HAVING A BABY AFTER 30

HAVING A BABY AFTER 30

ELISABETH BING and LIBBY COLMAN

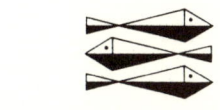

THE NOONDAY PRESS
Farrar, Straus and Giroux
NEW YORK

Copyright © 1980 by Elisabeth Bing and Libby Colman
All rights reserved
Published simultaneously in Canada by Collins Publishers, Toronto
Printed in the United States of America
Originally published in 1980 by Bantam Books, Inc.
Noonday Press edition, 1989
Second printing, 1989

Library of Congress Cataloging-in-Publication Data
Bing, Elisabeth D.
Having a baby after 30 / Elisabeth Bing and Libby Colman.
p. cm.
Reprint. Originally published: New York : Bantam Books, 1980.
Bibliography: p.
Includes index.
1. Pregnancy in middle age—Popular works.
I. Colman, Libby Lee.
II. Title.   III. Title: Having a baby after thirty.
RG556.6.B52   1989   618.2—dc20   89-7823

Table of Contents

Introduction by Donald Sloan, M.D.   ix
Preface   xiii

Chapter 1:   DELAYED CHILDBEARING   1
    The Phenomenon of Delayed Childbearing   1
    Who Delays and Why?   6
    Medical Considerations   13

Chapter 2:   THE PREGNANCY   30
    The Meaning of Pregnancy for Older Expectant Parents   30
    Special Concerns of Older Expectant Fathers   37
    Special Concerns of Older Expectant Mothers   42

Chapter 3:   BIRTH AND THE EARLY DAYS WITH BABY   51
    Birth   51
    Feelings for the Newborn   60
    The Early Days with Baby   67

Chapter 4:   SPECIAL CONCERNS OF THE FIRST MONTHS   78
    Breast Feeding   78
    Sex   89
    The Post Partum Blues   93

Chapter 5:	THE FATHER WHO HAS WAITED SO LONG	109
Chapter 6:	MOTHERING AND WORKING	122

    Staying Home with Baby   124
    Working Part Time   130
    Working Full Time   137

Chapter 7:	TIME FOR MORE?	147

EPILOGUE   150

MY STORY
    by Elisabeth Bing   151

AND WHAT IT MEANT FOR ME
    by Peter Bing   161

A FEW REMARKS
    by Libby Colman   165

Bibliography   167

Index   171

Acknowledgements

First and foremost we wish to acknowledge our debt to Arthur D. Colman, M.D. It was he who first suggested that we collaborate on our earlier book, *Making Love During Pregnancy*. He was an advisor and an inspiration through that project as through this. His wisdom and experience in the area of the psychology of pregnancy have been indispensable to us both.

Grace Bechtold at Bantam books has worked with us diligently and beyond the call of duty.

Several other people have contributed help and advice along the way, most especially Mervin Freedman, Ph.D; Verneice Thompson, Ph.D; Sarah Gray, R.N; Alan Moss, M.D.; Mary Moss, R.N; and Carol Fones, R.N, C.C.E.

We cannot acknowledge the individuals who contributed the most, those who shared their lives with us. We hope they recognize their own experience if not their own words echoing through these pages. This book is by them and for them; we hope it rings true to them.

Introduction

I am certainly prejudiced in favor of women who decide to have their babies after the age of 30, because if my mother had not done so I would not be here now. My mother, you see, was considered quite "elderly" to be giving birth to a child at a time when she was somewhere in her late thirties—her exact age being one of the things she used to keep secret—and I can remember being told stories at family gatherings about the chiding she took from her family and friends for having a child "so late in life."

My own history has helped me in my work as an obstetrician and gynecologist to reassure many women over 30, or even over 40, that they can feel comfortable in facing the world and their friends and families, whose culture and customs may have conditioned them to view late childbirth as unacceptable or deplorable. Myths and old wives tales seem to surround the idea of late childbirth.

I am happy to be part of a movement that is bringing new light to this subject. Thank you, Elisabeth Bing and Libby Colman for making use of your expertise and experience in the world of childbirth to add to this awakening.

Having a Baby After 30 deals with a very human problem of a scientific nature. My own medical training, as well as that of most of my colleagues, has certainly sharpened my scientific acumen, but often it has been deficient in providing for concrete medical situations. As the authors of this book have shown, the decision to have a child when the mother is over 30 years old cannot, in the vast majority of cases, be made solely on an abstract basis.

Much of what we know about the whole creation process is based on statistical analyses and results. These studies often mislead us because of the multitude of factors that are likely to crop up when we have to confront a real situation. So many cases never seem to fit the pattern we had been taught or that we had anticipated. I remember a wise teacher of mine saying that the very last area to be conquered in medical science will be the one involving creation itself. It seems as though a higher power is saving this knowledge for itself, knowing full well that it would be too much for a mortal to bear.

There exists an enormous dearth of knowledge concerning human emotion and the portions of the brain that regulate psychological events. We can't experiment with this aspect of the brain, and in fact only become aware of it when it does not function well. We know of it by its malfunctioning, that is, the occasional havoc it produces in our lives. Pregnancy is clearly one of the most profound psychological events in a human life. It is the ultimate psychosomatic experience.

Pregnancy plays a vital role in our culture. It demands social, marital, and emotional adjustments. Moreover, since the physiology of the female is uniquely adapted to it, women who decide to postpone childbirth to a time when it is culturally not entirely acceptable feel an additional burden. A normal event thus becomes fraught with pressures.

If pregnancy is considered normal in early years, if it is thought to be a symbol of female adequacy, anxieties are easily understandable when pregnancy is postponed to a period in life which seems "too late," or culturally unacceptable to many people. When physicians or parents become caught up in these cultural pressures, they are apt to fall back on the kind of "book knowledge" that reflects a mechanical point of view. And if science fails to answer all their questions, people often begin to function out of ignorance and fear. There seems to be nowhere else in medicine where the skills, attitudes, and feelings of the persons involved will be put to as great a test as when a couple approaches parenting late in life. If ever a doctor and patient needed to communicate, it is here.

I recall an incident, among many, that revealed this to me. A woman approached me for her first consultation. She was 40 years old, though her appearance and manner made her seem considerably younger. "I think I am pregnant," she started saying. "My husband and I want this baby very much, but my family is very upset that we are starting on our family so late in life. My mother even told me she felt herself too old to be a grandmother." She was obviously hurt that her own mother would actually try to deny her the right to have so important an experience simply because the time schedule did not coincide with her mother's concept of when things ought to happen. I spent a great number of hours with her and her husband in an effort to reinforce the validity of their own position, as against the social forces which they were attempting to reject—forces that tried to shape their lives according to extraneous factors. It was a challenge to me as a physician to learn so much about the psychological needs of this couple, to understand the intricacies of outside pressures and how they affect the patient's needs. And I wondered how the medical profession can learn to be aware of and deal with the emotional concerns of the people who come to us for what at first glance only seems to be purely medical and physical advice.

The answer to my question is really simple. It is you, the reader, the parent, the consumer, who will teach the doctor a new attitude. Your doctor is a tradesmen, and his medical school is a trades school, where he learns the skills and arts of his profession. These skills are made available to the public on demand. However, it is the reader, the consumer, who installs new attitudes and feelings in the doctor and thus changes his actual performance.

Pregnancy is a physiological process which embraces all aspects of human achievement. It is a normal process; it is nature itself (the root meaning of the word "nature" means *birth*); it is a somatic event. The body undergoes changes which have to be dealt with. It is an emotional event. Bringing another human being into the world, and being responsible for rearing it, involves a profound transformation of the psyche. And finally, pregnancy is a cultural process which is influenced by our religions, our families, our friends, our neighbors, our enemies, and even our history.

If you approach your pregnancy with confidence when you are 30 or over, you will convey this confidence to the hospital staff, your nurse, your doctor—in short, to everybody you come in contact with. I think we are moving rapidly towards a demystification of medicine, as a result of the dialogue that has already begun between the consumer and the medical profession. This dialogue will be of great service to the profession.

As for yourself, the reader, it is not good enough to yield to prejudices and social pressures. Pregnancy and parenting over 30 can and certainly should be an especially healthy process. Your belief that this is so will radiate from you, and those around you will bask in this radiance themselves. A new feeling and understanding will be created.

Read *Having a Baby After 30*. It will make you realize that it is not so late, after all!

DONALD SLOAN, M.D.
New York City
1979

Preface

Many people have asked us to write this book. Damaris Rowland was the first. Working as assistant editor of our book, *Making Love During Pregnancy*, she asked, "What is it like for women who delay having a baby until after 30?" Since then we have heard the same question asked over and over again. People who are pondering parenthood turn to us and ask, "What is it *really* like?" or "Should we or shouldn't we?" Sometimes they wish they could get pregnant by accident to take the decision out of their hands, but they have been too successful for too long at using contraceptives to let themselves get away with it. They want guidelines for making one of life's truly irrevocable decisions. They also want to hear what the experience was like for people such as themselves, people who were independent adults for a decade or more before becoming parents, people who had ten years of freedom and travel, people who had established careers. They have gotten used to a lifestyle that is free of children, and they are not sure that they will be able to adapt to the changes that would come with a baby.

Since the last generation bore their babies so young, there are not many women around who can tell others what it was like to raise children after a delay. Even more noticeably, since few mothers of the last generation combined careers with motherhood, there are few models for the typical young woman of today who expects both to work outside the home and to raise a family—and perhaps to have the work come before the family. Many women reach 30 and want to have a child or children, but have no way to know what it will be like to start raising a family after a decade of freedom. They may also be concerned about whether or not it is possible for them successfully to fulfill the dual role of mother and career woman. They hear that it can be done, but they are not sure how.

In our respective capacities as childbirth educator and psychologist, we see many pregnant couples and new parents. We asked them to tell us what it is like to delay having a baby until after the age of thirty so that we could write a book for others like themselves. The response has been overwhelming. Many couples have written us letters, from two to 25 pages long, describing their experiences. Others have shared their experiences in taped interviews conducted during the pregnancy and through the first year of their child's life. All of these informants have known that we were writing a book to let others know what the experience is *really* like. They have opened their lives to us and to the readers of this book. They have shared their joys, their fears, their life histories, their dreams for the future. They have told us how they decided to have a baby at this point in their lives and what they wish they had known before they started. This book is really their book. We are trying to summarize all we have heard from the many men and women who have shared so much with us. We will let them speak in their own words much of the time, for they are the experts. They are inside the experience. They are the ones who can best answer the question, "What is it really like to have a baby after thirty?"

1

DELAYED CHILDBEARING

The Phenomenon of Delayed Childbearing

After World War II, the average young American had a dream that he or she tried to make come true. It was the suburban dream, the dream of economic prosperity and family "togetherness," the dream of having a house with a yard, a husband with a job, and a wife with two or more children. After the disruptions of the war, it seemed that there could be no better life than that defined by love and marriage. Men and women tried to live up to this ideal by marrying young and producing babies immediately. The men were good providers and the women expressed satisfaction in giving up their jobs to get married or to have a baby.

By the mid-1960's, the dream had changed. The babies of the post-war period, who had been raised in the "suburban dream," were now adults. They created a new dream of their own, a dream that manifested itself in part through various "liberation" movements. When this generation came of age, the emphasis was not on stability and family, but on revolution and freedom. Men rebelled against the "gray flannel" image of the '50's, let their hair grow, and often "dropped out." Women rebelled against the "helpmate" image of their mothers and chose careers and birth control over white picket fences and baby bottles.

These dramatic changes did not take place in a vacuum. We could look for their roots in the psychodynamics of a generation raised by commuting fathers and lonely mothers, or in the economics of a society confronted by a ballooning population reaching the age when it would enter the job market at a time when positions were scarce and inflation zooming. In addition to the possible psychodynamic and economic explanations, we could turn to the expanded technology and availability of birth control as a factor in the changes. The pill was developed in time for the '60's. Soon afterwards, sex education moved into the schools; the IUD was introduced; abortion was legalized; condoms could be displayed and sold openly. Whether these were causes or symptoms, widespread contraceptive information (and effectiveness) created a situation that had never existed before.

It is true, of course, that a good number of women used contraceptives before this date. The diaphragm was in general use, and any woman who had the means could buy such a device after she had been fitted by a physician. However, it was only in the 1960's that people such as Dr. Alan Guttmacher fought for the law that permitted city hospitals to give contraceptive information to all clinic patients; that is to say, to the lower economic strata. It was, therefore, really the first time in history that large numbers of women of childbearing age learned how to exert control over their own reproductive organs to prevent or curtail unwanted pregnancies.

Every generation has had some women who delayed childbearing until they were over 30 or 40. During the 1930's many women put off having a baby until after the disruption of the war. But never before have so many women been so effective in not having babies until they wanted them.

The baby boom began in 1945. The babies born in

that year turned 30 in 1975. Enough of them chose not to bear children in their teens or twenties to cause a significant dip in the national birth rate. So many people of this generation decided *never* to have babies that national support groups were started for nonparents. In addition to groups in favor of having *no* children, there are now groups, such as Zero Population Growth, that encourage people to have no more than two well-planned children.

It is now turning out that many of the people who caused the dip in the birth rate were delaying childbearing rather than deciding to have no children. They are having their first babies in their thirties or even in their forties. This trend is apparent from the statistical surveys that have been done.

In 1960, wives aged 18–25 had an average of 1.4 births per thousand while wives aged 35–39 had an average of 2.7 births per thousand. In 1974, wives aged 20–24 had only 0.8 births per thousand while wives aged 35–39 had increased their birthrate to an average of 3.1 per thousand. In other words, there has been a definite shift towards delayed childbearing among married women in the United States since 1960. Fewer women are having babies in their early twenties and more are having them in their late thirties.

The trend towards delayed childbearing has been paralleled by two other trends, that of having fewer children and that of spending fewer years in the home as a full-time housewife/mother. Instead of marrying at 20, having the first of four children by 23, and expecting to see the last child off to school fifteen years later, an average woman today marries at 23, does not have the first of two children until after she is 29, and expects to see the last child off to school only five years later. Childbearing is viewed as an interlude rather than as a lifelong task.

Most couples will probably continue to have their first baby in their twenties. This is the decade of life in which men and women establish themselves as adults. Becoming a parent is accepted as part of becoming grown-up. Couples in their twenties feel mature enough to take on the responsibilities of parenthood, yet still feel young enough to deal with the physical strains of bearing and raising children.

There are still social forces at work which stipulate that one's twenties are the "right" time to have babies. Some people believe that it is medically dangerous to have a baby after the age of 30. Others feel that it is socially inappropriate to be "old" with an infant. Many feel intense pressure from parents and peers to produce offspring early. Many couples report being made to feel uncomfortable by remarks of family and friends, such as, "Now that you're married, when are you going to have a baby?" or, "Now that you've bought your house, when are you going to have a baby?" or, "When are you going to give us a grandchild? We're not getting any younger, you know, and neither are you."

We have talked to many women in their early and middle twenties who told us that they didn't know exactly when they were going to have their first baby, but that they were sure it would be before they were 30. Over and over again we heard 30 mentioned as the magic age. We have also found, however, that as women get closer and closer to 30, they find reasons to reevaluate their situations. As a woman of 29 told us:

> I never really decided to have children until I saw my 30th birthday looming up before me. Suddenly I felt that it was "now or never!" Up until that time it was just something I thought I'd decide about some day. For the past few years I've been sort of creeping up on a "yes" decision to have children, but I always thought, "Well, first I have to give up smoking, lose 15 pounds, paint the kitchen, or get further in my career." Then I remembered something my

dentist, of all people, told me: "There is never a good time to have your teeth capped, have a baby, or buy a house." I think there are very specific problems associated with having children at any age, and you can't say any one set of problems is any worse than another.

This woman, like many others, saw 30 as a critical threshold. At 29 she realized that if she were to have her baby by 30, she would have to get started immediately. Suddenly she saw her life in a new light. She became particularly worried about her marriage. Was it stable enough for children? Could she and her husband bear the strain? Would the romance go out of the relationship? Was he really the man she wanted to have as the father of her children? If she decided that he was not, would she still have time to find a new relationship and start a family before her biological time clock ran out?

Menopause does impose an upper limit on a woman's childbearing years. A man can change his mind about having children at any time. A woman who puts off the decision for too long will find that it has been made for her. Most women know that childbearing becomes more difficult, and then eventually impossible, as they get older, but it is not too clear to them at exactly what age these difficulties occur. When they approach 30, women want a very clear idea of exactly what to expect from their own bodies. Having waited so long, they want to know what is possible. Can they put off having children until they are 35 or 40?

As we will see in the last part of this chapter, medical considerations do not become serious until the late thirties. Thirty itself is not a magic age at which childbearing suddenly becomes more dangerous or more difficult. There is no cut-off date that separates "young" mothers from "older" mothers. Many investigators begin with the age of 35 in discussing the special concerns of women having babies in their late thirties and forties. We decided to talk with women in their early thirties as well because we felt that if they had been living independent lives without children for ten years, they would be subject to many of the same experiences as women in their late thirties.

We have found that the decision-making process often becomes extremely difficult for men and women who have avoided having children until the age of 30. It is easy to say, "I want to have children some day." It can be very hard to say, "I want to get pregnant now." In the next section, we will look at the experiences of some people who have delayed childbearing. What were their reasons for not having a baby in their twenties, and what are their reasons for deciding to have a baby later?

Who Delays and Why?

Most of the women with whom we spoke planned their pregnancies. Some became pregnant accidentally, through the failure of their contraceptives, but in these cases (at least for first-time mothers) the decision not to abort involved a conscious acceptance of the pregnancy and a positive desire to become a parent. Almost all of the people we interviewed who had their first child in their thirties or early forties *wanted* to have a baby.

We also spoke with women who would have had babies in their twenties if they had been able to conceive at that time. But we found that even when it was not a conscious choice, the fact of being older first-time mothers brought women into a shared experience. Even if they had wanted to become mothers in their twenties, the fact remains that they stayed in the work force longer.

Women who have their first child in their thirties or forties tend to be well-educated and to have good jobs. They are members of the middle class. After all, they have had time to establish themselves, to go back to school, to put away savings, to make the downpayment on a house. Even if they came from a background of poverty, they have moved up and are doing well.

Throughout this book we will be talking about the jobs and careers of the women who delay childbearing. This does not mean that all of them are "career women" in the sense of being highly committed to getting ahead in their jobs. It simply means that by the time a woman is thirty, if she has never had children, she is usually a person with a well-established work identity. If she started out as a teacher who expected to give up her job to start a family, but didn't meet the right man until she was 29, she has had time to establish seniority and to acquire a specialty credential. Even if she thinks of her work as "just a job," she is earning a formidable salary—and she is used to supporting herself. Even if she expected to stop working and stay home and raise her family, she will find that she has become accustomed to the work world and to her salary. Similarly, if she started off by just "dabbling" in painting or photography, or if she took a few courses "for the fun of it," by the time she is 30 she is likely to be taking these pursuits quite seriously.

The situation of a woman who becomes more serious about her career than she expected is typified by Connie, a corporate executive who had her first baby when she was 34. As she told us:

> I grew out of the secretarial pool. I remember distinctly being in an office as a secretary after I graduated from college. In walked a fellow who had been my lab partner in biology. He was the corporate attorney, and I was just a typist! At that point, I made up my mind to start achieving in the business world.

Connie actually got married and tried to have a baby in her mid-twenties, but she did not succeed in getting pregnant. She divorced and found that her job was more important to her than before. She remarried and became pregnant in her early thirties. It was a very different experience than it would have been ten years earlier. She was well-established and had a lot of contacts. She quit her job and started a business of her own, picking up clients gradually as her baby grew older and more independent. She would not have had such freedom (or such knowhow) as a member of the secretarial pool.

A secretary, a flight attendant, or a waitress may not be a "career woman" in the same sense that a physician, a college professor, a lawyer, or a corporate vice president is a "career woman," but many of the considerations are the same. Having a baby after the age of 30 disrupts a well-established pattern. The woman has to add the identity of "mother" to her ongoing sense of herself at a time when she is well past the formative stages of adolescence and early adulthood.

Men have always expected to have careers and to be parents. They may anticipate some conflicts between the two roles, but they generally see their career aspirations as part of their parental role of being providers for their families. More and more women are sharing the role of provider. Their salaries are not just for "extras," but establish the couple's standard of living. The Women's Liberation Movement has encouraged women to view their own careers as being equal in importance with those of their husbands. It is inevitable that such women will experience conflicts when taking on the responsibilities of motherhood.

Most of the women with whom we talked were married and had been living with or married to their husbands for several years (often more than five) before they got pregnant. This means that the couple had had time to establish themselves and to get used to a life pattern based on two incomes. The economic realities of inflation make it unrealistic for most families to expect to live on one income. Older couples are used to getting along quite comfortably. Many of them describe exotic vacations and a lifestyle that includes an active social life, frequent nights out, and a generally free and joyous time. A baby is much more disruptive to the lifestyle of such a couple than to one that takes on the adjustment to parenthood at the same time as the adjustment to marriage.

We also talked to several women who decided to have a baby even though they did not have a partner. We frankly expected to find more single mothers than we did. The overwhelming majority of women told us that they would not have done it on their own, that they wanted to share the responsibility and create a traditional family. The single woman who feels that it is "now or never" for her will find that we do not address ourselves to some of her special problems. She may have more trouble with childcare and with job conflicts because she does not have a mate, but she will also not be under the same pressure to accommodate to a changing marriage at the same time that she is adapting to the baby.*

The most common motive for postponing pregnancy, however, is to advance a career. Increasingly, women want to get established in their chosen field before having children. They feel that this will give them more options, more control over their lives. Once they have established their careers, they feel that they will be able to take off a few years without fear of "losing touch," or that they will be able to work out part-time arrangements. They may be in a position to become self-employed and thus in control of their own schedules, or they may have become so indispensable to their bosses that they can expect to have their de-

---

*See the Bibliography at the end of the book for suggested reading about single parenting.

mands met. They also may expect to be making enough money to afford domestic help.

A doctor or a lawyer is still very young professionally at the age of 30. After four years of college, three or four years of graduate school, and one to three years of apprenticeship work, the fledgling professional will be at least 28 before she is on her own and ready to think about having a family. We talked with an archaeologist who spent her twenties traveling, as part of her training and her initial work in her field. She was not ready for a stationary academic job until she was in her thirties. The same time-schedule applies for most academic disciplines.

Some of the best-known women who delay bearing their first child are performers. Singers and actresses must generally spend years working long hours for low pay before they receive recognition and get established, before they can risk taking a break in their careers. Dancers and athletes experience an even more intense pressure, for they live with the knowledge that they will reach their peak at an early age. They do not want to take a year out of their prime, and they know that they may be ready for retirement in their early thirties. As one such woman told us:

> I wanted to dance until I was thirty. We didn't consider our early thirties as "late" because most of our friends are older than I, not married yet, or married but having no children. In the performing arts, work demands extraordinary time, often twelve hours a day, to say nothing of tours. Our friends who did attempt to raise children under these circumstances are now divorced.

Not everyone who delays childbearing can explain her reason for doing so. Many women told us that they simply did not feel "ready" earlier. This usually means that they were not ready to settle down. They saw their mothers struggle with the burdens of the housewife/mother role, and they decided they would rather seek freedom and adventure before settling down. Many of these women were seriously searching for a firm sense of "self." They did not have a clear career direction and weren't sure what they wanted to do. They wanted to experiment with jobs, with sexual relationships, and with lifestyles. A typical woman of this kind describes her feelings:

> When I was 22 or 23, I decided I would wait until I was over 30. I just thought I wouldn't settle down until then. I've always known I wanted children, but by the time I was ready to seriously consider it, I decided to put it off until I felt—less itchy, you know? I just wanted to be free to move around where I wanted to go. I went to Europe twice and moved to a lot of places. I found I could get work wherever I went because I had had a government job and there are government offices in all the major cities where I wanted to live. I'd work for a while, then move on to another place.

So far we have discussed positive reasons for postponing childbearing, reasons related to personal or professional growth. There are also some negative reasons for not having children. These are related to the fear of becoming a parent. In sociological terms, they are the concerns for over-population, pollution, and other ecology related issues. On a more personal level, both men and women may fear parenthood as a trap, as something to be avoided at all costs.

Women who have established a clear work identity may never have thought of themselves as mothers. They don't think of themselves as nurturing types, and may have trouble imagining themselves taking care of an infant, puttering around the house, or driving school-age children in car pools. When they marry and have a mature, established relationship with a man, they are sometimes surprised to find themselves wanting children. It is not unusual for a woman of this kind to be afraid of losing control of her life. She does not want to be financially and emotionally dependent on someone else. She may also be afraid of having an infant dependent on her. Some women express this as a fear that they will not be able to give enough to their children. They have trouble imagining what it would be like to be a mother. They know what it is like to be a working person and what it is like to be in a family as a child, but they may have had little experience with women who have been competent both in their careers and as parents. They are afraid that they may have to give up all that they have worked to acquire. As they move into their thirties, these women may feel increasingly ready to invest personal energy into deep relationships, and may feel ready, for the first time, to make the commitment to have a child. One such woman says:

> The main reason I'm having my first baby at 35 is because I never had a realistic chance to have a baby before this. It took me this long to grow up and this long to have a situation that would welcome and nurture a child. I had a lot of living to get under my belt, so to speak, in my twenties. I got married only two years ago and now I'm going to have a child. It never could have happened before this.

After the age of 30, men and, especially, women may realize that it is "now or never." If they had previously decided that they didn't want a family, they have to reassess this decision now, for they are facing their last chance. Often, they decide that they are now mature enough. If they saw marriages ruined by children, or if they felt that their own parents were unhappy because of the burdens of children, they may have reached the stage in their own lives where they nevertheless feel that they can have a family without falling into the traps that destroyed others.

We have found that the men and women who postpone having children assess their lives very thoughtfully and make considered decisions about becoming parents. The answers that they come up with are not simple ones because the problems that they are contemplating are complex. Those who decide to have their children in their thirties or later seem dedicated to the idea that parenting must be done well if it is done at all.

For most people, the postponement of children involves factors such as job status, economics, the desire for a few more years of freedom, and the desire for a more stable marital relationship. Even though there are now many people who delay having children, the slightly older mother may still feel like an anomaly. She may be acutely aware of the differences between her situation and that of her friends who had children earlier. But when she weighs the differences, she is likely to be happy with her own choice. One of these women told us:

> Having reached the ripe old age of forty, I feel I'm in a position to really sit back and savor this. I've seen the limits to the satisfactions of a career and feel ready, and without a sense of sacrifice, to devote a lot of time and attention to my exceptionally well-tempered child without giving up my career obligations entirely.

Medical Considerations

A woman who is thinking about whether or not to have a baby later in life generally realizes that there are special concerns that come up for women of her age, concerns that become more intense with the passing years. Even though she feels as energetic and healthy as a woman of 28 or 29, the extra years may have caused some changes in her body that may affect her ability to have a healthy baby. These are serious concerns to thoughtful women, so we will try to clarify what they are and what role they may play in an older woman's experience of the childbearing years.

Many doctors consider 35 to be a crucial age at which there is likely to be a sudden increase in the need for special obstetric care. Sidney H. Kane, M.D., writing in 1966 for the Foundation for Medical Research in Philadelphia, stated that "advancing age in the primigravida (a woman having her first baby) would appear to produce certain inherent risks." But he continued to say that "the concept of the arbitrary age (35 years) at which maternal risk increases should be abandoned as a myth, and the more logical concept of a sliding scale of difficulty should replace it." All the studies we have come across have actually used a five-year scale, and they indicate that while the risk of some problems does increase with age, there are no precise, fixed conclusions about the rate of medical complications at each point. In most cases, it is more accurate to consider the age of a woman in relation to her well-being, her lifestyle, her general health, and her feelings about herself, her body, and her pregnancy. If she is in good health, her chances for a good pregnancy, a normal birth, and a healthy baby are virtually the same as those of a younger woman. A few genetic problems are clearly related to age irrespective of general health, but again there is no one year in which the risks suddenly increase. The rate of some problems accelerates with age.

To a great extent, the concerns of women of 30 and over are the same as those of any pregnant woman. Problems can and do occur at any age, but the vast majority of women have excellent pregnancies and give birth (without undue difficulties) to perfectly healthy babies.

Nevertheless, pregnancy is a time of extreme physical and psychological change. It is understandable that the medical profession, as well as those women concerned, should pay special attention to all the things that could possibly go wrong. We know that women who delay childbearing want to have a clear idea of the possible consequences of their choice, so we have decided to present a brief outline of the problems that are more likely to occur in the case of the woman who is having her family at a slightly later stage of her life.

FERTILITY-RELATED ISSUES

Possible Effects of Long-Term Use of the Pill or the IUD

A woman of any age may have difficulty conceiving after being on the pill for a period of time. She may not menstruate for up to six months after she stops taking the pill. Many physicians advise women to discontinue the pill a few months before they try to become pregnant.

The IUD (or Intra Uterine Device) has also been suspected of causing difficulties in conception, according to fertility specialists.

The longer a woman delays childbearing, the more likely she is to have used either the pill or the IUD, or both. We cannot give precise statistics because it is often difficult to ascribe infertility to a single cause. Women who have trouble conceiving in their thirties often had trouble when they tried to conceive in their twenties as well. A certain number of women who become mothers in their thirties would have had their first baby sooner if they could have. This influences the statistics on the ease of conception among women having their first child in their thirties.

The pill and the IUD do not seem to have created

insurmountable problems of infertility for the majority of women who have used them.

Physiological Factors Connected With Aging

As with other natural functions, fertility declines in both men and women with increasing age. Although a man produces fresh sperm continuously, his sperm become less effective as he grows older. Sexual activity may also decline with age, which can obviously affect fertility, since greater frequency of intercourse is likely to increase the odds of conception. The egg's ability to become fertilized is limited to a period of about 24 hours within a woman's menstrual cycle.

Follicles, the precursors to the ova (eggs), are developing within the female fetus before birth. After puberty, the follicles have matured and the ovaries will start to release the stored ova at ovulation during each menstrual cycle. Fraternal twins may result from the release of two eggs at the same time, whereas identical twins are caused by one ovum splitting in half and then developing simultaneously.

The older a woman gets, the greater the possibility that she does not ovulate each month, and thus the less chance she has of becoming pregnant. If she does ovulate and fertilization does occur, there is a greater chance that cell division may not proceed normally.

Age also increases the possibility of accumulated traumas in the uterus or the fallopian tubes, such as fibroids or infections, as well as possible injuries to the testes. Fortunately, the reproductive organs in both male and female are located in very safe places and are not easily injured.

Part of the reason we hear more about fertility problems among couples over 30 is that they feel pressed for time. A younger woman may stop using contraceptives but take no other steps towards conception than her usual lovemaking. She would also feel more comfortable going through time-consuming tests should they be necessary. A woman who is over

30 years old, particularly one who is over 35, has generally set herself a deadline and is more likely to feel anxious to have her baby as soon as possible.

MALFORMATIONS OF THE FETUS

Possible Age-Related Causes of Malformation

According to Sylvia Hay and Helen Barbano in their studies of "Maternal Age and Birth Order on the Incidence of Selected Congenital Malformations" (*Teratology*, 1972), "it appears certain that the risk of some malformations is increased among births to older women." But they also point out that studies seem to vary a great deal and that many have shown no correlation between maternal age and malformation in the infant. In their own work, it became apparent that most of the malformations occurred in women over 40 years of age.

Other studies have shown a higher incidence of problems in women over 40. Some birth defects are caused by a dysfunction in the chromosomes of the egg or sperm. Sometimes the irregularity is so severe that the fetus cannot survive and is spontaneously aborted. Other times the defect is so slight that the child can develop normally or with only a slight problem.

The egg released one month may for some reason have damaged chromosomes, but the next one or the next ten may be fine. The fact of having produced one defective ovum neither increases nor decreases the odds of producing another. A genetic counselor can advise a particular couple what their odds are for creating a healthy baby.

Down's Syndrome

Down's Syndrome (also known as mongolism and trisomy 21) is the best known and most common of the genetic problems that occur among older parents.

Statistics show that for women who are 20 years old, only one in 2,300 births will be affected. For women between 30 and 34, the rate is one in 750, while for women who are 39 years old, the rate climbs dramatically to one in only 280 births. Among women between 40 and 44 years old, the rate again increases to one in 130 births. Finally, in women over 45, one in 65 will be affected. These are the facts of the risk rates. Given these statistics, it is up to the individual couple to decide whether or not its chances of producing a normal baby are good.

Down's Syndrome is determined by the condition of the #21 chromosome in the particular egg and sperm that create the fetus. Other congenital abnormalities (such as Kleinfelder's Syndrome and Turner's Syndrome) are created by problems in other chromosomes. A chromosome may be defective for various reasons. In some cases, the problem is passed from generation to generation. This does not seem to be the case for Down's Syndrome. The most widely held theory about the cause of this particular problem is that the chromosomes do not separate correctly during cell division before fertilization.

Modern medicine does not know how to prevent or cure Down's Syndrome, but it has learned how to detect it and many other genetic defects before birth. A fetus carrying a serious chromosomal problem can be aborted. Unfortunately, an older woman has a greater chance of carrying such a fetus and also has less time in which to conceive again.

Detecting Malformations by Means of Amniocentesis

Amniocentesis is a test performed to detect the possible presence of genetic diseases such as Down's Syndrome and other chromosomal abnormalities. There are special centers in which a woman can have the procedure performed and also receive genetic counseling to help her understand the meaning of the test results.

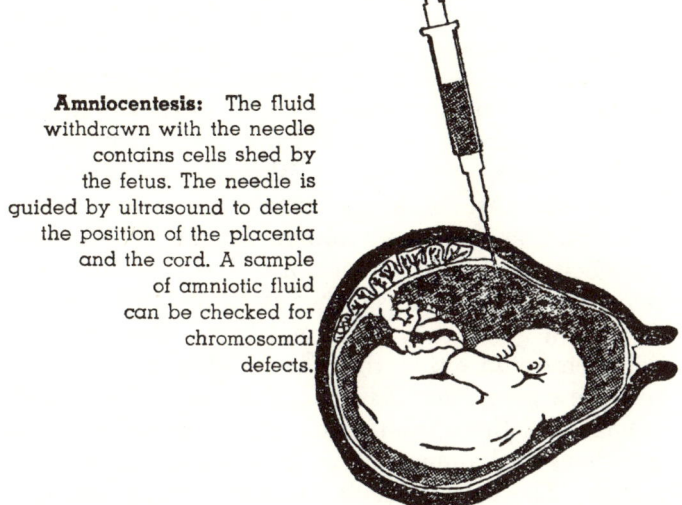

Amniocentesis: The fluid withdrawn with the needle contains cells shed by the fetus. The needle is guided by ultrasound to detect the position of the placenta and the cord. A sample of amniotic fluid can be checked for chromosomal defects.

Amniocentesis is a procedure for obtaining a sample of fluid from the woman's womb. This can be done without disturbing the baby because of techniques for determining the exact position of the placenta and the fetus within the uterus. First, a sonogram is taken. Sonograms operate like radar by beaming high-frequency sound waves whose patterns change according to the density of the objects through which they pass. These patterns can be projected onto a screen or oscilloscope. They show the exact position of the placenta and fetus at any given moment, and the physician can gently insert a needle into the uterus at a safe place where the baby is curved well away from the uterine wall. A little amniotic fluid is withdrawn. It will contain some cells that have been sloughed off from the fetus. These cells contain the exact chromosomes of all the cells in the developing baby's body. When they look at the chromosomes, the laboratory technicians can tell whether or not the baby has Down's Syndrome or some other genetic defect. They can also tell whether the fetus is a boy or a girl. We have found that some couples are eager to learn the sex of their baby, but others prefer to be surprised at the birth. Of course everyone wants to know that their baby is not carrying any discernible genetic defects.

There exists a calculated risk with any procedure, but in the case of amniocentesis the risk is slight. Therefore, an informed woman will be able to make the decision of whether or not to have the procedure performed on the basis of her statistical risk of giving birth to a genetically abnormal baby. The procedure will determine either that the baby is normal or, in some few cases, that it is defective—in which case the woman has the option of having an abortion. Those who have had amniocentesis done tell us that it is not painful. The most difficult part may be the long wait for the result, which currently takes from three to five weeks. This can be a very anxious time for families who have reason to believe the fetus may have a problem.

The knowledge that a fetus is healthy far outweighs the dangers of amniocentesis for those parents who do have reason to suspect a genetic abnormality. Nevertheless, this, like all medical procedures, should be reserved for cases of genuine risk and should not be performed to resolve idle curiosity. It is generally recommended for all women over 35, or for those who are known to have a genetic problem in the family.

Amniocentesis is not being used as widely as was hoped when the procedure was originally developed. This may be due in part to a lack of publicity in popular magazines; it may be due also to a natural reluctance of parents to face the possibility of genetic difficulties or to the widespread feeling among women that they would not want to undergo an abortion even if they learned that there was something wrong. It is important for doctors and midwives to inform prospective parents of the option of amniocentesis, and to refer them to genetic counselors if necessary to help deal with the medical and emotional implications of the test.

OTHER CONCERNS OF PREGNANCY

Fears and Anxieties

Some matters may be of more concern to the older woman, but generally her worries and anxieties are the same as those of younger mothers-to-be. Although we have no statistics to offer, we suspect from our experience that there is a slightly greater tendency for older women to be anxious about the well-being and normalcy of their babies than their younger counterparts. This may be because they have heard that older women are more likely to have problems or because they have simply lived more years and are more aware of the things that can go wrong, not only in childbearing, but in life generally. They are less likely to have the magical optimism of youth. A pregnant woman at any age is likely to focus all of her worries on the new and unknown force in her life, the baby. The fear that something may be wrong with the baby may take precedence over all her other concerns temporarily, or it may actually repress them.

For some women, pregnancy is a placid and blissful time. Many other normal, well-adjusted women are filled with fears and anxieties. The hormonal stimulation of the pregnancy and the excitement of creating a baby can give a woman a feeling of very special well-being. Many women, older as well as younger, feel physically and emotionally better during pregnancy than they had for years.

Miscarriage

Miscarriage is such a well-known problem of pregnancy that it is often taken lightly, at least by those who have never experienced it in their own lives. In actuality, miscarriage is a difficult event, especially for a woman who has had trouble conceiving or is worried about having a baby before too many years go by.

The deepest impact of miscarriage is often emotional. When a woman has delayed childbearing and finally decided to have a child, she is often impatient to "get on with it." She may have trouble waiting to conceive again. The temptation is to try again right away. Women are wise to wait for a few months, however. There is a lot of grief involved, even in the loss of a fetus in the earliest weeks of pregnancy. In addition to the emotional considerations, miscarriage creates physical problems, especially weakness from the loss of blood. A woman who rushes into another pregnancy may suffer from anemia and fatigue.

A miscarriage is an event that takes its toll on a woman's body as well as her emotions. It is likely to be more discouraging for a woman over 30, but it is serious at any age.

Fatigue

The older woman is likely to be more easily fatigued. She may feel a lack of energy, especially in the very last weeks of pregnancy or in the early weeks after the delivery. But there is no norm for this. Fatigue is probably more closely related to nutrition and general health than to age. Fatigue during pregnancy may be due to a woman's lifestyle, her occupation, or her activities.

If people of 40 tire more easily than people of 30, it is often because they lead more sedentary lives. In a few sports that require exceptional flexibility, strength, speed, or stamina, such as gymnastics and swimming, age can be a deterrent to excellence. Even 25 is considered old in these sports. Forty is old in most professional sports, but for amateurs the story is quite different. There are seventy-year-old tennis players and even marathoners; if there are not many, this is because so few undergo the necessary training, not because more couldn't do it if they wanted to.

The physical demands of pregnancy and birth are different than those of a football game or a basketball game, but good muscle tone is equally important. In childbirth, the most important muscles are in the back, the abdomen, and the perineum. Sports and childbearing both put a strain on lung capacity and on the heart. Most midwives and obstetricians advise a sensible exercise program for pregnant women of all ages to get them in shape for the event. Those who lead sedentary lives may have to work harder to prepare for the unaccustomed stress.

Minor Complaints

Backache, varicose veins, constipation, and nausea are all common complaints of pregnancy that may be increased by age, but few women suffer unduly from any of them. Obviously, one's physiological capacity is slowed down somewhat with the years, but there seems to be no significant increase in discomfort during pregnancy among older women. There are some illnesses that an older woman is more likely to have than a younger one, among them diabetes and degenerative illnesses such as arthritis and cardio-vascular disease.

Toxemia

Toxemia is a syndrome rather than a disease. As a complication of pregnancy, it involves any of the following symptoms:
- Hypertension (high blood pressure)
- Edema (swelling caused by retention of water

in body tissues, especially noticeable in hands and feet at the end of the day)

- Weight gain (especially a sudden gain after the 20th week of pregnancy caused by water retention rather than by the growth of the fetus or extra calories consumed by the pregnant woman), and
- Excessive protein in the urine.

The word "toxemia" means "poison in the blood." Actually, we do not know what causes it. We *do* know, however, that it is more likely to occur in first pregnancies, among diabetics, in women carrying more than one fetus (i.e. twins or triplets), and in extremely young women (under 16).

Toxemia in pregnancy is serious because it can lead to pre-eclampsia, which has such symptoms as headaches, trouble with vision, mental dullness, and abdominal pain. At its most severe, it becomes eclampsia proper—convulsions that require immediate delivery of the baby to save the mother and child.

Fortunately, the advanced stages of toxemia are unlikely to occur among women who receive adequate prenatal care. The early signs—high blood pressure, edema, weight gain, and protein in the urine—can easily be detected by tests routinely performed on pregnant women at office visits.

A nutritious diet and regular check-ups are especially important for pregnant women of any age who have high blood pressure or other reasons to suspect toxemia.

LABOR AND BIRTH

Preparation For Labor

Labor is not necessarily more difficult for the older woman. Statistical correlations indicate that there seems to be remarkably little difference between younger and older primiparas (women giving birth to their first child) in length of labor or ease of expulsion, although there is an increased incidence of caesarean births.

Many women and men in the United States prepare for childbirth by participating in classes that teach either the Lamaze or some other method. These classes train the mother to function with as little medication as possible during labor and delivery by controlling discomfort through breathing and relaxation techniques. The reason for this is that anything ingested by the mother is also ingested by the baby. The classes also give men and women a chance to learn how their bodies function. The same techniques that work at birth are also helpful in other situations of stress. If there has been any decrease in muscle tone as a result of age, the exercises that are learned and practiced in childbirth preparation classes will help remedy the situation before the birth.

Rh Incompatibility

The Rh factor is a substance found in the blood of almost 90 percent of all Americans. In itself, it is not affected by the age of the mother. However, the discovery of Rh incompatibility may affect the older woman's decision to have a baby.

People who do have the Rh factor in their red blood cells are called Rh positive (Rh+). Those who do not are called Rh negative (Rh−).

Rh negative blood reacts to the presence of Rh positive blood by developing antibodies that attack and destroy the red blood cells that carry the Rh factor. Rh negative blood can be sensitized and made to form antibodies through transfusions of Rh positive blood, but since the dangers of incompatibility have been recognized, this rarely occurs.

An Rh positive woman does not have to worry about danger to herself or her babies. An Rh negative woman only needs to be concerned if she carries the baby of an Rh positive man, for such a baby has a 50–50 chance of being Rh positive. Sample blood tests are routinely taken on pregnant women. If an expectant mother is Rh negative, her husband is also tested. If he is Rh positive, a sample of fetal blood is taken to determine the Rh type of the fetus.

When an Rh negative mother carries her first Rh positive fetus, she does not generally become sensitized and develop antibodies. When the placenta detaches from the uterine wall at the birth, however, fetal blood generally does pass into the mother's system. Her Rh negative blood will begin to develop antibodies to destroy these incompatible red blood cells. An Rh negative mother who gives birth to or miscarries an Rh positive baby is treated within 72 hours with Rhogam, an anti-Rh gamma globulin that will prevent her blood from becoming sensitized. If she were not treated, any subsequent Rh positive babies she might carry would be in danger. The antibodies from her blood could pass through the placental barrier into the fetus's system and damage its red blood cells. The baby's life would thus be in danger unless the condition were detected and treated.

When an Rh incompatibility is detected, the mother's blood can be monitored to detect the possible development of antibodies so that corrective measures can be taken. In extreme situations, the baby may have to be delivered early and receive blood transfusions immediately.

Caesarean Births

Among older women, approximately 25–30 percent of all births occur by Caesarean section. The incidence is only 10–15 percent among women under 30. The national percentage used to be about 4–6 percent twenty years ago. Many doctors now feel that it is safer for the baby to be born abdominally than vaginally if the mother has a prolonged labor, a possible pelvic disproportion, diabetes, or other medical indications (such as dangerous Rh incompatibility or advanced eclampsia as described above).

The muscle tone of the uterus of an older woman may be less flexible than that of a younger woman in some cases, and therefore less able to expel the baby. Older women are also more likely to have developed general health problems that affect the course of labor. However, we know that the statistics for older women are adversely affected by the inclusion of some over-thirty women who have developed medical problems after many pregnancies. The healthy first-time older mother is still a relatively unfamiliar obstetrical phenomenon. We suspect that this contributes to a general tendency among obstetricians to be more conservative when dealing with older women and to be more likely to perform Caesareans than with younger women.

Some doctors feel that improved surgical procedures make it possible for Caesarean births to have few complications. It should be kept in mind, however, that a Caesarean is a major operation, associated with all the risks, problems, and discomforts of surgery.

It is frequently beneficial for the baby if the mother goes through some labor before the Caesarean because the uterine contractions seem to "massage" the baby's chest and in this way prevent respiratory complications in the newborn.

Caesareans may be performed with either an inhalation anesthesia, such as nitrous oxide, or a regional anesthesia, such as a saddle block or an epidural block. If there is a chance that a Caesarean may be necessary, a couple may want to discuss types of anesthesia and types of incisions with their obstetrician. They may also discuss the possibility of having the father present throughout to provide comfort during the procedure if the mother has a regional anesthetic.

There are several good books about the Caesarean experience for families who are anticipating or have undergone this operation.*

---

*See the Bibliography at the end of the book.

POST PARTUM

Recovery

Recovery from childbirth seems to be more related to the nature of the delivery and the general health of the mother than to age. A woman who has had medical complications will have more trouble recovering than one who has not. Similarly, a woman who is generally tired and run down will recover more slowly than one who is physically fit. While we feel that it makes sense that older women should recuperate more slowly, we have not seen much evidence of this among the women with whom we have talked.

Menstruation

A woman will resume menstruating, if she does not nurse, approximately four to six weeks after giving birth. There seems to be no difference at all between older and younger mothers in this regard. As long as a woman ovulates, her menstruation follows certain patterns, whether she is 25 years old or 35 years old. If a woman breastfeeds, she will generally not menstruate until she weans the baby, though it may happen, occasionally, that her period will return while she is still nursing her baby.

Contraception

It is wise to discuss the method of contraception with the physician after the baby is born. Breastfeeding does not necessarily mean that a woman cannot become pregnant, though the possibility is less than if she does not nurse her baby.

Coping with New Demands

The demands of the first few postpartum weeks amaze almost all new parents. Women seem particularly surprised at how much time it takes simply to care for the baby and for their own personal needs. Some women have an easier time coping with such demands than others.

Although a few older women are impatient with their infants, we have found that most are able to find solutions for their problems. Older women have had more experience in coping with stress and change. They are also often more financially secure than their younger counterparts, and can therefore afford help more easily.

Books, articles, and organizations are springing up to support men and women who think their lives might be richer and better without offspring, but this is still not the ideal for most. In spite of the growing evidence that children make marriages less happy, interfere with work, and take huge amounts of money, the generation of the post-war baby boom still expects to bear babies of their own—when they are ready. As one woman said:

> I read every book I could find devoted to the subject of whether or not to have children, and bored poor John to death by discussing the subject endlessly. We were both well aware of the drawbacks of childbearing. But somehow, all along, I knew deep down inside that the tremendous happiness I'd feel in loving another human being as much as I knew I'd love my child would make the experience worthwhile. And how right I was!

2
THE PREGNANCY

The Meaning of Pregnancy for Older Expectant Parents

Pregnancy has many meanings for different individuals. The feelings of a given individual will often be complex, and sometimes contradictory. As we talked to expectant parents and read the reports sent to us, we often felt amazed at the avalanche of feelings a single person tries to cope with. The men and women we spoke to described their attempts to understand and sort out the various feelings that they had about their situation. They wondered about the effects it would have on their lives in the near future.

For many, pregnancy seems to be a time of introspection, a time for reevaluating the past and making a commitment to the direction their lives will take in the future. It calls into question values and assumptions about family life and personal identity. It suddenly brings up memories of childhood and of past family relationships.

The meaning of pregnancy is shaped both by the individual's experience of family life in his or her own childhood and by the experience of adult life prior to the commitment to have children. Men and women over 30 have already had a decade or more of living independently in which they have established their own style, which may be only partially compatible with their upbringing. They need to find patterns that will fit both their new identity and their honest feelings about families they grew up in.

Pregnancy seems to convey the meaning of a whole new life for many people. Most obviously, of course, it means a whole new life for the baby who is being created. It may also carry the hope for renewal for the rest of the family. This may be most powerfully true in a planned pregnancy that has been awaited for a long time.

The birth of the first child certainly brings a radical change in lifestyle, especially to a woman who has been working. This change can be feared or it can be eagerly anticipated. Many women have told us that the whole adventure seemed like "starting a whole new lifestyle." During pregnancy, this was exciting, even wonderous. One mother-to-be said, "Maybe I'll be a totally different person. I don't really know what to expect."

We have been struck by the number of people who choose to have a baby when they are ready for a change in their own life, when they feel ready to move into a new phase of their own development. Some people who find that they cannot get pregnant choose another avenue of change. We have known several women who quit their very secure jobs in large corporations and started their own small businesses when they were told they could never get pregnant. Others started law school, dropped out for a while, or in some other way changed their careers entirely. A certain number of these women who make a radical change in their careers then get pregnant unexpectedly and find themselves in the middle of *two* whole new projects simultaneously. However the details work out, pregnancy and having a baby create upheaval. It is not unusual for a couple to choose to conceive when they feel ready for some kind of new direction in their lives.

The meaning of pregnancy as a life change is reflected in the large number of real life changes that are often precipitated by a pregnancy. Perhaps the most common is that of moving into a larger or simply a "better" home. Career changes are also common. It is logical that this should occur for mothers and fathers who want to create time to stay at home to care for the infant, but career changes also occur among parents who do not expect to do much direct childcare. It seems to be part of the general upheaval to try to be generally bigger, better, and more secure in order to fulfill one's own concept of what it means to be a "good parent." A new trend we have noticed among women is a tendency to change their names during their childbearing years. This generally means starting to use their husband's surname instead of their maiden name, although it may mean giving up the surname of a first husband and returning to a maiden name.

The idea of creating change in one's life by having a baby might not be altogether acceptable, as it appears to put the interests of the parents above those of the child itself. We think, however, that such feelings have a very positive value, at least during the pregnancy and early weeks of the baby's life when it does not yet have or need an identity of its own. A parent who is ripe for change will be more ready to set aside time and energy to devote to the care of the baby, and will be less frustrated by the inevitable disruptions caused by the baby.

Often the people who are most conflicted about having a baby are those who want no disruption of their established lifestyle. Rather than being delighted with the opportunity to move into a new phase of their own lives, they are afraid that they might be forced to accept an identity that they do not want.

Pregnancy creates some real changes in life, but sometimes the anticipation of change can be more dramatic than the change itself. Men and women who are eager to experience a "new life" may be those who enjoy the experience the most.

Young adults are often committed to creating a life for themselves which will avoid what they perceive to be the mistakes of their parents. Such a commitment may be easier to carry out before they become parents themselves. Pregnancy may challenge the manner in which they have adjusted. The couple can use this period of waiting to consider the meaning of parenthood and to wonder what the future will be like.

There is both an imaginary and a real side to this process. The child is still a fantasy. Its demands have not yet been experienced; its cries are still unheard. The prospective parent does not know how he or she will react. One woman told us the following:

> It's nice to wonder about what you are going to produce. We have musical genes on each side, so we wonder if our offspring will be like our mothers, completely non-talented, or like our fathers, musical. One of the anomalies of my husband's appearance is that he has speckled eyes. Will we have a child with polkadot eyes? Then you will know; it's the kind of thing that you will know was created by the mixing of the protoplasm. It will be a blending of us!

Many people feel a special closeness in the marriage during a wanted pregnancy. "It has been a positive thing for us. We are much more aware of our bond together." In fact, the pregnancy can be so ideal that a woman is not eager for it to end:

> I almost don't want the baby to come because things are so neat between us. We have never been so close. We have been working toward this, I feel, but we are *so* close and *so* supportive and *so* giving to one another. I can never re-

member us being so willing to make ourselves vulnerable to one another. We've worked really hard at it. I think pregnancy has brought out a lot of caring. I finally broke down and allowed myself to feel dependent and to admit I need him, and a lot of maternal things that I've denied before, I'm allowing to come out now. He's benefitting from that, he's getting it.

At the same time that the abstract issues are being contemplated, the waiting period may be used for practical things that need to be done. The baby will need a place to sleep and the family will need an adequate income. They might have to rearrange their house or even their lives to make room for the baby and provide for its care. These are the very down-to-earth changes that have to be made. There are dozens of books that give advice about the layette; magazine advertising informs the expectant parents about baby equipment; but who is there to give advice about the larger issues related to personal identity?

Expectant parents who do not intend to pattern their lives after those of their own parents may be in a quandary as to whether the advice they receive is compatible with their own values and expectations. For the couple who have delayed childbearing, this often means wondering how to anticipate an overwhelming transformation without knowing many other people who have come through it in a way they respect or admire. They may be eager to have a child and feel "ready" for a change. They may be mature and competent adults. And yet they are on the brink of the unknown. This may be exciting and threatening at the same time.

Pregnancy makes many people aware that, fundamentally, they are aging and moving into a new developmental phase. They feel that they are becoming a member of the older generation, that they are turning from being simply someone's son or daughter into also being someone's father or mother. They become acutely aware of new responsibilities and may feel suddenly older and more mature as a result.

From a distance, it may look as though some people grow smoothly through this transition from one phase of adult life to another. They seem ready to add another dimension to their lives, a dimension that brings a new meaning to their existence as well as new commitments and extra work in their everyday activities. They seem to be looking forward to parenthood as though they can't get there fast enough, especially when they have been waiting so long.

There may be some people who really are in the enviable position of being so ready for parenthood. We have generally found, however, that when we get a closer look, even those who seem to pass easily through this transition are experiencing doubts. Most people seem to find it a rough passage.

In spite of having made a conscious decision to become a parent, the imminent reality may create uncertainties and anxieties. Pregnancy is often a time when men and women suddenly ask: "What have I gotten myself into?" "Will I really be able to cope with this?" Even though they had chosen to take the step, they may have intense moments of doubt which seesaw back and forth with moments of elation. They had been enjoying the pleasures of adulthood unencumbered by the ties of family.

When women are heavy with child, they may panic because of their memories of the problems their parents had. They may recall the innumerable books and articles about mothers who have felt abused and restricted by their role, and fathers who have deserted their families. They may fear that as parents they will be burdened with incessant interruptions and demands, with arduous tasks that inhibit "personal growth." They may seem to momentarily forget all the positive emotions which led them to the decision to have a child.

It may be frightening to face inevitable change without having any way to really know what the new life will be like. Vacillating between the emotions of optimism and despair is understandable and even to be expected under the circumstances.

The following passage is taken from a man who explained his reasons for delaying parenthood:

> I wanted to postpone the birth of our first child for as long as we did (six years) for a number of reasons. In the first place, I have always found aging distasteful, particularly because I cannot do anything about it, and having children just seemed like another indication of one's advancing age. Hence I was anxious to postpone having a child. Second, Mary and I had a comfortable lifestyle. After a number of years of marriage, we had learned to live fairly nicely with one another, and I was not certain I wished to alter anything we had achieved. Third, I felt that having a child before I was as certain as I could be that our marriage would remain intact would be foolhardy. I wanted our child to have two parents to grow up with.

The same views might have been expressed by a woman. The fact that they were expressed by a man shows that the sexes share many of the same concerns and that both take parenting very, very seriously. Nevertheless, there are some issues which seem to be more commonly experienced by men than by women. First we will look at what men have told us about how they relate to pregnancy. Later, we will look at the feelings of women.

Special Concerns of Older Expectant Fathers

One of the most striking features of men's reactions to becoming fathers is their concern about being economically responsible, not only for themselves, but also for their wives and children. This seems to take on special meaning when the wife has been working and contributing to the family income, a situation that is particularly common among older couples. The man may experience the loss of a sense of security and wants to take on an extra job. Even if his wife intends to continue in her career, the man tends to regard his own financial responsibility as central to the role of fatherhood. This economic involvement is so deeply ingrained in men in our culture that it still predominates, even after the years of exposure to the theories and realities of women's liberation.

> Here I am at the age of 47 and a father for the first time. I'm still getting used to it, but I am behaving just like the cliché of a new father. After Linda became pregnant, I still had mixed feelings about it. I'd be facing an awesome new responsibility; my lifestyle would be restructured drastically; all rather selfish feelings. I also worried about job security, etc. I was also aware that a new adventure awaited and that we would have a child to carry on for us.

At 47, this man was certainly older than most new fathers, but his concern both for economic security and for the meaning of his child as a continuation of his own life, his own family, is not unusual. Confronting a birth, especially at a more mature time in the life cycle, brings the parents to an intense awareness of their own mortality, and this in turn gives rise to a desire to make sure that there is a continuum, that they have produced something of their own that will live beyond them. In this way they are participating in the renewal of life, not only for themselves but also for the younger generation. Through the ages, this aspect of parenthood has been mentioned by poets, politicians, and philosophers. Aristotle went so far as to say that the most natural act for living beings was to produce other beings like themselves and thereby participate in the eternal and the divine. While this abstract notion may not always be kept in mind during the daily demands of parenting, it is often the source of a man's deepest feelings about discovering the meaning of becoming a father.

Participating in these universal rhythms may not be a completely happy or easy experience for a man. If he has struggled to break away from his own father, and has worked hard to establish himself as a different kind of man than he perceives his father to have been, he may also want to be a different kind of *father*. He must feel very secure in his own identity to be sure that he is not losing ground by becoming a father. He may wonder if he will inevitably become just like his own father, or whether he will be able to hold on to the style that he has fought to achieve in his own adulthood. Will he be able to remain integrated while coping with the demands of caring for a son or daughter, or will he find himself re-creating the family patterns of his own childhood, patterns he may have rejected, but still may fear?

The pull back towards one's own childhood experience is very great when one is creating a child of one's own. Family life takes on a new perspective, but old memories rush forth and even become dominant. The patterns and values of one's formative years follow one through adult life. When there has been a hard-fought struggle to free oneself from the patterns of the past, whatever balance has been achieved may be thrown off by the new conditions created by the transformation into parenthood.

> Both Jane and I were terrified to be like our own parents. It happened to both of us. Our parents were really like children. My father was egotistical. He never seemed available when I needed him and wanted to spend time with him, and it terrified me that I would be like him and resent my own child.
> It seems quite clear to me now that I'm not looking for my child to fill my own inadequacies, and now I don't feel I'm like my own parents. I still have my own life and the baby is not an invasion. It's all pluses. I was afraid the baby would be demanding and take away my own space. But what is happening is that I am getting something. I'm not denied anything. That was really my biggest fear. People never seem to tell you those things about having a baby.

The ability to confront the older generation as a father as well as a son is a struggle for some men but not all. Although older fathers may often be men who have postponed parenthood because of their reluctance to become like their own fathers, there are also men who become fathers in their thirties or forties who hope to follow the family patterns. Perhaps they were late in establishing themselves in their business or profession, and feel that it is important to be settled and secure before starting a family. Perhaps they did not meet a like-minded woman until they were older. Whatever the reason may be, instead of being afraid of being like their own fathers, these men are proud and happy to be like them and carry on family tradition.

The family is not the only formative influence on a person's values. Peers in high school and college may be particularly important in establishing assumptions about how to live out adult life. Some of the men and women who postpone forming a family experience themselves as distinctly different from the peers of their younger days. Others feel that they are living up to expectations, that they are acting out values shared by others.

> I remember after graduating from high school that one of my classmates got married within one year. At the time I thought that was astonishing. At that age you see yourself as moving along, doing and accomplishing things together. You really tend to find a small, intimate circle of, say, ten people, which comprises your inner circle. You tend to judge yourself in terms of this intimate group, and you follow each other closely, playing a game of leading or following. What you accomplish has a lot to do with what they accomplish, and at that time we were accomplishing things at quite a clip, considering we were busy working our way towards college and good jobs. So when one of us stepped so precipitously into marriage, even before or just as he was entering college, I must admit it was a shock. In fact, it was a very creative thing to do, but just as you tend at that age to rely on information from your peers to ease yourself over one hurdle or another, you also sometimes quite inexplicably do something totally on your own. He seemed to have done that with no help from his friends. He was the first. And of course after that, as the years passed one after another, people got married and had families and our circles expanded and became more varied. And so most of our group had either formed their families while they were in their twenties, or there were a few like myself who more and more, and for different reasons, drifted into a satellite position to what we were sure was the

general trend. Therefore, I became, or took on, the role of friend, godfather, and slight eccentric to their children.

This man experienced himself as going against the trend by postponing marriage and parenthood until his late thirties. At the same time, he was very happy with his special status. He felt that his life was exploding and expanding in every way. He had urges along the way to have a cosy family life, and when he finally did marry, he happily assumed that he and his wife should have children.

Other members of this generation who delayed childbearing may have responded to their peers in a very different way. Not all saw family life as the normal trend. In contrast, they felt that one was *not* supposed to have children.

We were brainwashed when we were in high school and college. Everybody talked of zero–population growth. They said: "Don't overpopulate, stop the bomb, dedicate yourself to improving the world, march for freedom, liberate yourself from traditional family and sexual patterns." Finally I realized I would have to have my own say about my destiny. I changed and started thinking by myself and the pressures seemed to diminish; I mean the peer pressures.

Parents and friends are not the only people who seem to influence the way young adults choose to live out their lives. Many look to someone outside the family or even outside their own personal acquaintance as a role model. For men, this often involves a meaningful relationship to a mentor, someone who may not only be important in advising the younger man in professional matters, but who may also provide an ideal for emulation in the personal sphere as well. A man may cling to the autobiography of a great man as an inspiration in both career and family life. Such models may be experienced very strongly because they offer reassurance to a person who wants to do things differently from either his own parents or his contemporaries.

Men are likely to feel isolated in their role as father. They seem rarely to discuss their family problems with other men. This situation may be increasingly true for women as well, now that they are spending their twenties fully engrossed in a career rather than in the more traditional role of being a mother.

Special Concerns of Older Expectant Mothers

The awareness of advancing age has certain connotations for women that it does not have for men. Women know that they cannot delay childbearing forever; if they postpone too long, they will come to a point when they can no longer bear children. What is at issue is not merely the problem of being older and therefore tiring more easily, but the irrevocable fact of menopause and the pressure this brings to bear on the timing of pregnancy in a woman's life. Many women would like to wait until they feel "ready" to have a child, until they have accomplished all that they wish in their career, until they feel that they can afford to take a "time out." But they also experience a conflicting need, the need to have a child "while there is still time," or "before the biological clock runs out." They may set themselves the deadline of 30 or 35 and then adjust it when things don't work out, but they sometimes continue to feel the pressure of increased probability of birth defects and also of wanting to be young enough to enjoy their children. Particularly for women who have not conceived as soon as they tried or who have lost a baby through miscarriage, the issue of pregnancy after 30 can be complicated by the feeling that this is the "last chance." However, as more and more women are choosing to delay, more and more of them are beginning to see 30 as their *first* chance to have a baby.

As we saw in the last chapter, many women no longer assume that they will marry and have children as part of their early adult lives. They may go through their twenties without giving it much thought. They may be surrounded by friends who are not having children either, or on the other hand, by friends who are having children but who are also making heavy economic sacrifices to do so. Many of them really don't think of themselves as "old" when they approach and pass thirty. They are finding support in women's literature for remaining childless, and they see their lifestyle as appropriate and admirable.

> I waited until now to have a child mainly because I didn't want a baby in my twenties. I was a tomboy as a child, not one to play with dolls, and I never felt terribly close to my own mother. I never thought much about having children as a teenager or in my twenties. I suppose being a tomboy contributed towards my lack of interest in children. In fact, I was always a little frightened of infants and could never imagine myself caring for one.

It is hard for a woman who has never thought much about having children and who has never spent much time around them to really imagine what it will be like to have a baby of her own. She may need to use the pregnancy to get ready for the change and to get used to the idea of becoming a mother.

> I'm hoping somewhere in the back of my mind that it is not going to be as difficult as it seems in the books. My pregnancy certainly isn't as

difficult. I haven't had anything. It seems a lot of the books build up to prepare the woman for the worst. I think it's going to be a lot of fun to be a mother, but I had to work through a lot of very negative things that I was picking up from the culture around me. There were the things I've read and the things I've heard, and then just things that came up inside my own head, questions like: "Don't you know couples that have kids are much less happy than couples without them?" and "What will happen to your career?" and "Do you know how isolating it can be to be a mother in this society?" Ninety-nine percent of the women I've been around in the past few years have not been mothers. The few I have known that have children are the wives of men that I work with. My only role models are women with no children at all or the absolute feminine stereotype that just freaked me out. Sometimes this whole thing feels like a leap in the dark. I feel a real need to talk with other women like myself before I have the baby, just to be sure it really can go well.

The excitement of finally being pregnant is tempered by some anxiety about how to combine career interests with mothering.

On the one hand I am blissfully happy. At the same time, because I'm older and have strong professional interests, I feel sad that I cannot give myself to full-time mothering. I will be superimposing this new life of childrearing on top of my old life of teacher and painter. In order to manage it, I shall have to hire part-time help at some point.

In her last month of pregnancy, a career woman told us: "Sometimes I wish I could just be a mommy like everybody else." There may be a positive pull in both directions.

Women who have delayed having children are likely to find themselves confronted by the incongruity between their professional or job status and their conspicuous family role. One woman shared with us her experience of pregnancy in an almost all-male world:

> At first, clothes were getting tighter, then there were only a very limited number of things I could wear, and then I was in a whole new wardrobe. You knew they knew. You knew they were looking at your stomach when you walked in, but people never said anything. I think they were very afraid. They didn't know if what they said would be considered sexist. But I don't think they are taking me less seriously because of the pregnancy.

Another woman we spoke to shared this feeling. She selected maternity clothes that were as consistent as possible with her usual style. She was aware that her condition made some men acutely uncomfortable, but that most were delighted with it. She found that other women, even at her level of management, were very supportive and excited for her. She received mixed advice, from "Keep on working or you'll go crazy," to "Why don't you just take off and enjoy your baby?" but she did not feel the pregnancy was a handicap at work. Her only embarrassment occurred when she tried to pull her chair up to the table at an important board meeting and found that her belly got in the way. She felt a little silly, sitting with her chair so far out from the table that she had trouble taking notes.

Women (and men, too) often really start to relate to the child during the pregnancy. They try to imagine what it will be like and they begin to establish their relationship to it. It seems like a fortunate rule of nature that pregnancy takes nine months.

> I haven't had my baby yet, so I don't know what it's really like. One thing I do now is think a lot about the sex of the child. I usually start by thinking about a little girl, because I think I am partial to having a little girl. We have had her name since the beginning, but haven't told anyone. We love her already. I think about reading to her, holding her, dressing her, sewing for her, cooking with her, taking walks with her, and sharing hobbies like painting and gardening and reading and animals. Then my mind switches to him, our little boy, whose name we also have, although we have two names that go back and forth. In very little time, I love him very much and I'm doing just as many wonderful things with him. Either sex will be fine. Like all parents, I want a healthy child (with perfect eyesight).

Just as men reevaluate their relationship with their parents when they are on the brink of becoming fathers themselves, women are also likely to have deep feelings about their parents at this time. They often find themselves reevaluating how they were cared for. Sometimes this means vowing not to do it in the same way themselves:

> As I watched my parents experience bitterness in their marriage, I came away thinking that what I could offer my own child was parents that were very much in love and parents who had strong interests of their own.

This woman would not have considered having a baby until she was sure that she was in a deep, committed love relationship with a man. She wanted to work to establish that relationship before adding the baby. Such an impulse is particularly strong among people whose parents were divorced. It also seems to hold true that the daughters of women who had few interests of their own seem especially likely to resent the intrusiveness and over-dependence of their mothers. They have vowed to live their own lives differently. Postponing motherhood is part of this vow.

Most of the women with whom we talked had mothers who were traditional housewives and who gave birth under medication, relied on bottles and formulas for feeding their infants, and raised their children according to schedules and rules. The women who have chosen to delay having babies seem particularly committed to prepared childbirth. They are informed of the processes of their bodies during pregnancy, wish to participate actively in the birth, expect to have their husbands involved, intend to breast feed the baby, and expect to differ from their own parents in many other ways as well. The specifics vary from family to family, but pregnancy seems to highlight the similarities and differences between the generations. The issue may be as simple and objective as the ability to hold a job:

> My mother had never been brought up to work, so when she got a divorce it was really a hardship on her. That's why she always encouraged my sister and me to get good grades and to train for a profession. I would never feel comfortable staying home all the time.

One of the fears of many women is that they will inevitably be drawn into replicating their own mother's style. They are afraid that in becoming a mother, they will become their *own* mother. Then they will be doomed to repeat the mistakes of the past.

Early in the pregnancy all I could think about was my own mother. She had children, and look what happened to her. Two different husbands, and neither one lasted after a baby was born. I had to remind myself that my relationship with Jim was different than that. I know I'm not like her, but I felt the old pull.

Women whose mothers were very unhappy may experience this anxiety most acutely:

Being a housewife means being a mother, and being a mother means being a housewife. I think one of the reasons I waited was that I wanted to work through those fears of being like my mother. I had a lot of fears of falling into that kind of trap, and I really did see it as a trap. I felt that if you went that route, that was it. That was all you could do and all you could be. It was very, very frightening to me. My mother is a very unhappy person, so my strongest role model for mothering was really terrible.

Women with happier relationships with their own mothers may react quite differently to the pregnancy. For them it may mean a new level of intimacy, a new kind of sharing. One woman told us: "I wish I had started to have children earlier so that I might have had more understanding of my own parents." Another described how much closer she and her mother had become since the pregnancy.

It is not unusual for women in their thirties to have gone through a period of rejection of their parents followed by a reconciliation. Many maintain that they would not have been as comfortable sharing the pregnancy with their mothers when they were younger because they would have been afraid that their mothers might take over. As older women themselves, they feel more secure about their ability to assert their own values and take charge of their own lives, and therefore they can afford to maintain a more tolerant attitude about the differences between themselves and their parents. We spoke to several women who had moved to other parts of the United States or even to other countries during their twenties, but had returned to the region in which they had been raised as part of the general settling-down that occurred in their late twenties or early thirties. We were surprised to find many couples in their thirties who were living within an easy commute of their parents. Most were interested in working out good relations between the generations at this time even when they were aware of conflicts.

Although spending a decade working in the outside world may not seem to be direct preparation for mothering, it may contribute to a positive philosophy towards family life and parenting. A woman may come to the realization that even the most glamorous job can become boring and repetitive occasionally and therefore less than completely fulfilling. Some women feel that they have lived life fully. One who was worried about what she had heard about the boredom of mothering said to us, "Well, if it gets dull, I'll just remember you can feel trapped at work, too. It can be a kind of pit or worse. I'd rather be trapped with kids and at least have had the experience."

At the beginning of this chapter, we discussed the meaning that pregnancy has for different individuals. Perhaps it is suitable to close it with a quotation from a woman whose own positive perspective on having a baby after 30 we have found to be shared by many other men and women:

> I think the joys of having a baby later come
> from the deeper appreciation one gains of all
> things from added maturity. They also come
> from doing something very much out of choice
> rather than having it happen to one. They come

from knowing one's own and one's husband's or wife's personality because one has had time to develop it, and then being able to appreciate the extraordinary fact that a baby combines you both into an entirely new person of his or her own. They come from being renewed when one is "ripe" rather than ripening. They come from the added pleasure that anticipation confers on a wish that is finally fulfilled.

3

BIRTH AND THE EARLY DAYS WITH BABY

Birth

Many of the things we will discuss in this chapter could apply equally to younger parents. We have worked for years with younger mothers and fathers, sharing their feelings of elation and anxiety. In working with parents over 30 years of age, we found a great many similarities as well as many differences in their reactions to becoming parents. Some of the differences are subtle. We have tried to put them down in this chapter as they were related to us, and we hope that many of the older parents can relate to the widely varying responses we found.

Since the moment of birth is symbolic of all beginnings, a manifestation of our deepest creative force, and the first moment of visual and tactile relating between parents and their children, it should be as wonderful as possible. When we talked to the older parents, we were struck by the intensity with which they experienced these first moments between parent and child. Seeing and then holding one's own child moments after birth, or actually helping to deliver it by gently lifting the baby under its arms out of the vagina, is an overwhelming experience, whatever the age of the parent. It may be, however, that the greater readiness of the older mother and father give these universal emotions an even more intense meaning.

It is our belief that prepared births are beneficial for the entire family. Childbirth education provides expectant parents with information and techniques that can reduce anxiety and make the whole period before and after the birth healthier and more rewarding for everyone involved.

It is not necessary to go into detail about what constitutes an exhilarating birth experience. The baby is ready to be born and adjusts smoothly to the outside world. The mother is ready to give birth; her body opens a passage and pushes the baby out. The father is ready to love them both and to celebrate his paternity. Together, the family labors through the strenuous physical part of the birth, and together relaxes in the joy that follows. When the experience has been postponed—for whatever reasons—the years of waiting, or thinking about whether and when to have a child, will make the moment of birth infinitely more awesome. In retrospect, parents refer to the event as "unbelievably wondrous," as "the most moving experience of my life," or, in a lower key, as "a typically exciting unmedicated delivery."

It is hard to find words to describe the event when all goes well. Parents remember what it felt like long afterwards. They remember their feelings towards the baby and their feelings towards each other, especially if they are lucky enough to give birth in a setting that allows them to stay together.

Increasingly, hospitals are recognizing the importance of allowing the family to remain close together during and immediately following the birth. Alternative Birth Centers with "birthing rooms" can be found in large and small hospitals alike. Different hospitals have different rules, but all of them share the assumption that a birth should be treated as a family event, not a medical event, unless a problem develops.

The age of the woman is often a factor in whether she is given the option of laboring and delivering in a birthing room. Some hospitals automatically define women over 35 as "high risk" cases. However, we have spoken with many women over 30 and even over 35 who were active, healthy, and well-nourished, and who were accepted as "low risk" patients in Alternative Birth Centers. Some had to transfer to traditional delivery rooms, but most gave birth in a birthing room.

Birthing rooms are usually located on the labor floor of a hospital in an Alternative Birth Center, which is simply a space that is designed to accommodate the family during labor and birth. It has a homelike atmosphere with carpets and drapes, gentle colors, a rocking chair, pictures on the wall, plants, and a comfortable bed. Such an environment eliminates the uncomfortable last minute rush from labor to delivery room. The woman can also give birth to the baby in any position that is comfortable for her and among people who make her feel secure. There are generally windows, adequate pillows, backrests, a TV, books, and a comfortable chair for the person (or people) who accompanies the woman in labor.

Such an arrangement can be truly family-centered. The father can often room-in, rather than being separated from his wife. Some hospitals provide a cot while others use a large double bed so that the father can share the room. The hospital can provide breakfast or other meals for both parents.

We feel that all labor rooms should have such a warm and gentle environment. Surely, the safety of childbirth does not depend on stark and uncomfortable furnishings, scrubbed walls and bright overhead lights. In a hospital setting, it can be extremely easy to move a woman from a family-centered room to one which is thoroughly equipped with the latest electronic devices if there is a genuine need.

More humane environments in hospitals encourage

many families to have their babies in a hospital instead of opting for a home delivery. The shift from the home to the hospital was introduced some 50 years ago for obvious medical reasons. Nowadays, however, when the public has been educated to understand the hazards and risks connected to childbirth, it has also been recognized that giving birth in a hospital should not necessarily imply giving birth in a stark and frightening environment. In fact, it has become evident that women labor better, that their anxiety levels are reduced, and that even the purely physiological aspects of birth function more smoothly when they are in comfortable environments and are not separated from those they love and trust.

Either the father of the baby or a close friend may accompany the expectant mother to childbirth classes to learn about the techniques to use during labor and delivery. A woman's companion will adopt the role of a "labor coach." He or she will be able to observe, correct, encourage, and generally support the mother during her labor. Nurses and occasionally doctors may undertake the role of coach, but the teamwork between the mother and her husband or a very close relative or friend is wonderfully effective and often far more emotionally satisfying than being coached and helped by a stranger.

Instead of creating an atmosphere in which the family feels like an intruder into medical territory, an Alternative Birth Center tries to make it as comfortable as possible. A woman with a two-month-old baby shared her experience of giving birth in an Alternative Birth Center with us.

> A friend had told me that having a baby was really going to change my relationship with my husband, really put a strain on it, especially when we had been together so long without a baby. But I have experienced it just the opposite

way. Ken and I have gotten so much closer. It started in the pregnancy, but it got stronger through the whole birth experience, having him there and coaching me. The best part was spending that night in the hospital bed together, which was just incredible. The baby was born at 10:30 at night. I didn't sleep a wink. I just stayed up all night long staring at him and staring at Ken. It was neat. It really drew Ken and me close together, unbelievably so. Our love for each other has really grown. Ken is wonderful with the baby and takes care of it a lot, especially in the first couple of weeks when I was still afraid to be left alone with it. It was Ken who was totally relaxed. He was the one to calm the baby at first. It has all been so fantastic.

For Kathy and Ken, the birth experience was an integrated part of the whole process of becoming parents. When all three came home from the hospital, they felt a very special closeness and excitement.

Ken took off a month from work and Kathy's mother came to help out for a week. By the time Ken returned to his job, Kathy and the baby were well adjusted to each other. Kathy remarked with surprise that she had continued to look pregnant to other people and had not been able to wear anything except her maternity clothes for several weeks. At first this had disturbed her, but then she realized that, in a sense, she was still almost as closely linked to the baby as she had been when she was pregnant. In her dreams she was still pregnant. She looked at her baby in wonderment:

> It's the most creative thing one can do, that one can produce. He's the one that I housed for nine months, and now here he is. It just sort of makes

everything else unimportant. I know I'll get back to those other things, but for now they seem so silly.

For Kathy the birth was not a single moment or even a single day. At 34 she was ready for this new experience, the process of creating a child. The time in the hospital was particularly intense for her, and it stood out in her mind as the period when she, her baby, and her husband were the closest they had ever been. It was for her the beginning of experiencing her family as an entity unto itself.

Unfortunately, there are sometimes circumstances that keep a birth from being exciting and positive. Sometimes these circumstances are social or environmental, sometimes they are psychological, and sometimes they are purely physical. Birth is far too complex and transformational an event always to be free from complications.

Not all births result in the most optimal experiences, but mature couples are able to deal realistically with the events they encounter. One advantage of being an older parent is this ability to cope with stress and adjust well to complications or disappointments. The sight of a healthy baby can usually compensate for a difficult or even an unpleasant birth. A woman who had experienced a hard time during the labor and whose baby was delivered with forceps told us:

> Giving birth to this new person and holding her in our arms transformed in a flash a state of fear and anxiety to one of happiness and fulfillment in us that is nothing short of a miracle.

The birth of a child is an event that involves the expenditure of a lot of energy for those who participate in it. Some expectant parents seem to spend as much time preparing for the birth as they do preparing for the baby. Some parents tend to view the birth experience itself as a personal test. The birth becomes a rite of passage that must follow a preconceived plan in order for the woman to feel that she is fully initiated into womanhood or motherhood. This is a very romantic, even a sublime, notion. Unfortunately, it sometimes leads to a profound and unfortunate sense of failure. A particular woman may believe that she has to suffer to prove she can endure; she may be terribly disappointed with an easy birth. Another woman may believe that she has to give birth easily and quietly and be able to pick up the baby and go about her business immediately if she is to be a "real" woman. For her, a difficult labor or a need to recuperate might be devastating emotionally. Either an exceptionally easy birth or an exceptionally difficult birth can damage the self-esteem of a woman who is using this moment to measure her worth.

By focusing too much attention on birth as an isolated moment, instead of viewing the experience as part of an ongoing process, couples can set themselves up for failure at a time when they need all their personal resources available for the challenge of parenting.

> I wanted to be superlady and have a fabulous, natural childbirth. I was very cool when I went into labor. I calmed my husband, joked with the nurses, refused all medication, even when I had bad back labor. I was so pleased when the doctor said I was 7 centimeters dilated and everything was fine. A few minutes later the baby's heartbeat stopped on the fetal monitor and I was rushed into surgery for a Caesarean.
>
> One part of me was happy to be out of the pain of back labor, but after the operation my fear and discomfort were enormous, and my disappointment was very great. Everything I had planned was changed. My thrill of seeing my

baby born had been denied me. I had had no chance to show how "brave" I was. I woke up with catheters and I.V.'s and surgical stockings. I was full of Demerol. Moving to nurse my child was terribly painful. I was totally involved with fears about myself and felt very disinterested in my baby. She looked totally unfamiliar, and I was jealous that she resembled my husband more than me.

This most unfortunate feeling of "failure" is often encouraged by doctors and nurses who talk about women who have prepared for childbirth as "successes" or "failures." Their point of reference seems to be that being administered medication equals failure. We have found it hard to convince the medical profession that failure or success are concepts which simply do not exist for childbirth. The preparation involved is a preparation for childbirth and parenthood, not a challenge to "make it" or "fail at it."

We have spoken with women who admitted that they were more involved with themselves than with the baby at first, and who had trouble "letting go" of the birth experience. This is hard to admit, especially for a woman who wants to be a perfect mother; it is a true and valid experience nevertheless and must be acknowledged. It seems most likely to occur among women, regardless of age, who have had a very difficult labor with real personal discomfort that required medical intervention, including separation from the baby.

Childbirth preparation greatly increases the probability of a happy outcome for a birth, but it cannot provide any guarantees. There may be no such thing as being "over-prepared," but there is such a thing as investing too much in the birth experience. It is important to deal with whatever problems occur by confronting the disappointment that may go along with them. Whoever is assisting in the birth should help to create a supportive and sympathetic atmosphere in which the mother will feel comfortable and secure.

Unfortunately, women, as well as their partners, often feel that preparation for childbirth guarantees a childbirth without much pain and with practically no help or medication. This feeling is indeed a great problem that childbirth educators, as well as physicians and nurses, have to deal with. We have frequently found that even though we never promise a smooth labor and delivery—our preparation classes are designed to provide information and knowledge and to teach relaxation and other techniques the couple will require in the difficult task of giving birth—most couples nevertheless expect to achieve a perfect childbirth. The hospital staff, on the other hand, whether wittingly or unwittingly, often imposes value judgments on a couple that has prepared for childbirth, according to which the mother's performance is measured in the unrealistic terms of success or failure.

Several women have told us that they did not experience any rush of "mother love" at the time of birth. Two said that they did not realize that they felt anything at all for the baby until they found themselves crying with compassion for the child— one when she heard him cry after a blood test, the other after the circumcision. In these cases the baby seemed to help draw the mother out of her feelings of self-pity. Some women may need more help than others in dealing with their feelings about a bad birth experience.

Any woman for whom aspects of the birth experience simply don't make sense, don't fit her image of how things ought to have gone, is likely to continue to worry about the birth and to feel inadequate or incomplete. It does seem to help to be able to talk out the entire experience and to try to put together exactly what happened as a first step towards getting on with parenting, of letting go of the birth experience and integrating it with the ongoing experience of life. A close, loving, and understanding family is perhaps the best help of all. A childbirth education class often has a reunion so that new parents can talk about these feelings.

We have found that women who have Caesarean sections are particularly likely to be still ruminating on the event months and even years later. They seem to benefit a great deal from a chance to try to understand exactly what happened and to reassess their own experience. There are special support groups to help women deal with these emotions following a Caesarean.

A good birth experience can be like a wonderful wedding ceremony—it can be a symbol of the great joy the entire family and even the community of friends take in the beginning of a new phase of a profound relationship. But a good birth does not guarantee a good parent-child relationship any more than a good wedding guarantees a good marriage.

Age has generally little to do with the difficulties of learning to live with a new family, though, as we mentioned before, the older couple is usually more prepared psychologically to adjust, and therefore better equipped to cope with a new life pattern.

Feelings for the Newborn

Research over the past decade has examined the question of whether "mother love" is instinctual or learned. By observing the behavior of many women with their newborn infants, scientists have identified a pattern which they call "bonding." Bonding, quite simply, is the unique relationship that is established between a mother and her infant in the earliest hours and days after the birth. It has been found that virtually the same phenomenon occurs with fathers when they have the opportunity to be alone with their babies.

Both the mother and her infant have been through a physically straining event. They had been physiologically united; suddenly, they must adjust to being separate. Their hearts, lungs, abdomens, and brains must get used to the new condition of physical separateness. These adjustments take time and seem to be accomplished most smoothly when the mother and child are able to see each other, touch each other, and hear each other as much as possible. Researchers have spent hours analyzing films of infants and their parents. They have found that the newborn baby responds favorably to the sight of a human face, the touch of a human hand, and the sounds of a human heart and a human voice. The mother spontaneously reaches out and caresses her baby's torso, his arms and legs, his fingers and toes. She puts him to her breast, offers him nourishment, and lets him hear the sound of her voice and the familiar beat of her heart. These initial moments are part of the process of getting acquainted. If they cannot take place soon after the baby is born, it may take longer for the mother to feel comfortable and sure with her baby.

Hospital routines used to come between parents and their children. Increasingly, obstetrical services are trying to make it possible for parents to be with their newborn babies as much as possible. The extra contact seems to help mothers respond more favorably in the very beginning and also to be more nurturing during the first year of the baby's life. Although a mother who has had a difficult birth experience may be very tired, she may also need to have her attention directed away from her own discomfort and towards her child. One woman described her experience this way:

I didn't feel anything for him at first. All I could think of was my own pain. When the baby was brought to me later, my feelings were a little stronger, and each time he came I started feeling something a little more. The hospital was encouraging me to have rooming-in, but I resisted. I was looking out for myself. The next morning I said I would hold him all day and nothing bad would happen to him, but they came in and gave him a blood test. I burst into tears and realized that my maternal feelings were really there.

When a woman does not have continuous contact with her baby, she may feel as though she has "lost" it and as though it is not hers any more. This may be especially true when the baby has to be put into the intensive care nursery. The mother may begin a process of mourning for the "lost" child and then have trouble reversing her emotions when the baby is discharged from the hospital and given back to her. Research, such as that done by Kennel and Klaus,* indicates that it is especially important for these families to be able to continue seeing and touching each other every day so that they continue to be familiar with each other and so that their love can grow. Klaus and Kennel also stress that the love of parents for their child can grow slowly and surely, and that the first skin contact after birth, though important, is not necessarily crucial to the relationship.

Even when parents are allowed to snuggle with their babies, there is no guarantee that mother love and father love will spontaneously emerge and remain constant thereafter. Parenting is a complex task that lasts the rest of a lifetime. Mothers and fathers can take very good care of babies from whom they

---

*See bibliography.

were separated during the first two weeks. Similarly, mothers and fathers can feel estranged from babies who have never left their presence. The word "bonding" has been used to describe a common phenomenon that pertains to the spontaneous experience of many mothers and fathers when they are with their newborn infants. Pediatrician Barry Brazelton has used the word "attachment" to refer to the rather more complex and long-lasting process of parental love. Bonding is a process of recognition and acceptance; attachment is a process of falling in love.

Many couples instantly recognize their child and love it totally. Others have moments of doubt, even when they have participated in the entire birth process.

> I was very excited when my first child was born. It had been a hard labor, but that was forgotten when I saw the little baby actually there. As soon as she was lifted up and I knew it was a girl, I leaned towards her to greet her. She was still dangling upside down, the way they do in the doctor's hand, and I was saying, "Rachel, hello," but then Alan and I looked at her and we said, "You're not Rachel!" They gave her to us to hold, and she wasn't Rachel. She was tiny and very fair. The Rachel we had had in mind was supposed to be nine pounds and dark. I felt her tiny body in my arms and looked up at Alan. We both knew she was Laura, and we loved her as much as we would have loved Rachel.

Although some parents report instant recognition of their own baby, the more usual experience is wonderment and a need to get acquainted, a desire to explore every inch of the strangely familiar and yet totally unknown member of the family.

She seemed like a tiny stranger, and I called her Baby for the first few weeks because her name didn't fit her yet. It shocked me that I felt so separated from a being with whom I had shared the ultimate intimacy and who was still totally dependent on me for her nourishment.

Bill and I discovered ourselves growing more and more attached to this little person who became Sarah. We were falling in love with her, and I can now say that if you take all the clichés about the feelings of parenthood and roll them together, you would be describing our feelings. I realize that to the rest of the world, Sarah is just another cute baby, but in my mother's magic eyes, she is the most beautiful and marvelous creature in the whole world.

As with all love relationships, the feelings between parents and their children are uniquely specific to the individuals involved. Sometimes the parents feel love at first sight. Often, the early days (or even the early weeks) are less intense. Sometimes the process may be very gradual indeed. A woman may feel that her baby is "just a blob" at first, and yet may take very good care of the child and grow to love it more and more with each passing week. It is easier to admit in retrospect that "I really didn't like him very much at first." At the time, such negative feelings are very hard to acknowledge because they contradict the ideal of being a perfect parent. In fact, however, feelings of estrangement can coexist with feelings of great love.

Family circumstances at the time of the birth can also influence one's feelings towards the baby. A woman who is worried about a bad relationship with her husband, or who is anxious about her career, or who is overburdened with housework, may not be able to relax and have the pleasure of falling in love with her baby. Occasionally what began as a very good relationship in the hospital becomes something quite different after the mother and baby are discharged.

> Then the homecoming! No one, not books or classes or anything, prepared me for the shock. I felt utterly helpless. I had never babysat, never been around small babies, never had any experience, and here this tiny creature was my charge! Being so weak from the birth, waking every four hours during the night for feedings, and being in a highly emotional state, nearly rocked my boat too far. Everything about caring for the baby seemed an enormous hurdle.
> But then she started sleeping through the night at five weeks. What they say about entirely breast-fed babies seemed to be true. She is lovely and healthy and a pleasure to care for. After two months, she seemed like a real person instead of an other-worldly creature, and began to smile and look upon the world with sparkling eyes. What seemed like an awful burden became great fun.
> And now I enjoy learning all the new things about her, learning to read her moods, how to put her down so she doesn't cry, taking her to parties, shopping, to the park. There is a constant development that makes her the most unboring, unrepetitive thing I've ever done, despite the fact of having read so many women's lib books calling babies drudgery.

Feelings about the baby go through many changes. The newborn *is* a stranger—and a very demanding stranger at that. Love may emerge only slowly. Even after parental love is well-established, it can be mixed with feelings of annoyance and even anger.

There have been little moments when I've been angry at him. I wasn't expecting that, but I'm not surprised. I just say, "Oh, you're making me mad, huh?" I'm feeling mad and I try to figure out what's going on and how to fix it.

This fairly objective attitude, which allows a new parent to recognize her feelings and try to change the circumstances that cause them, seems to help make childcare easier. A mother who blames everything on the baby will have a hard time finding solutions because babies are very hard to control. For example, a mother who says, "She lets me sleep a half hour and then demands me again," will continue to feel angry and frustrated. Another mother in the same situation took quite a different view of things:

The other day we went out and I got tired, but I said, "When we get home I'll be able to sleep," but when we got home I couldn't go to sleep because he was needing me again, and I was a wreck, physically so exhausted I could hardly deal with him. I had just pushed myself too far, and him too. There were too many adjustments for him, getting in the car, being with people; he was exhausted, too.

While neither mother liked caring for a crying infant when she was overtired, one blamed it on the baby and the other accepted responsibility for the circumstances and assumed that the baby, like herself, was responding to events that she could modify.

Feelings about the newborn are almost certain to be intense. Mother love and father love do not always begin immediately. They may require time and acquaintance, a period of "getting to know you." Birth is a brief moment of transition, but the entire post partum period (literally the time *after the separation*) is also transitional. Everything is new and strange. It brings out the wonder and anxiety of the unknown in all of us, whether we are younger or older parents.

The Early Days With Baby

Many animals seek out a private and secure place to give birth. They respond with rage if they are disturbed. Rats and mice may even eat their own babies if the nest is disrupted during the critical hours. We must be very careful about making generalizations from other species, but this sensitivity to disturbance which is characteristic of many other mammals around the time of birth is also experienced by some women. Humans do not have to rely exclusively on their primitive instincts, but they are nevertheless under the influence of biological forces. Many expectant mothers experience a desire to "prepare a nest." They want to make sure that everything is ready for the baby, and they want to feel secure in the fact that the environment that they have prepared is safe for the birth. They also want to remain as undisturbed as possible afterwards.

We were quite surprised to find the desire for "nesting-in" to be particularly strong among older women. We had expected them to want to continue their full lives and return to their careers. Instead, we found that many women we talked to were extremely happy not to have to go straight back to work. They wanted to spend the next weeks or months with their baby—although they generally assumed they would eventually rejoin the work force. One said:

> I was not sure what would happen after the baby was born, whether I would want to rush back to my work. But I soon found out, to my utter delight, that this particular period can be a

most creative one in life. Men or women who have had no children can never really sit back and assess what they have done. I did just that, and wondered what I would now do with the rest of my life. I could do this pondering while I was thoroughly enjoying my time with my baby. But in the long run, I know that full-time mothering is only a temporary job.

I feel almost sorry for men that can't take out this period in their lives to think about themselves, take courses in other fields, and not have to rush into obligatory activities.

Shakespeare refers to "the childbed privilege . . . which belongs to women of all fashion." This "privilege" is a period of removal from the hustle and bustle of the everyday world, and it is prescribed for women after childbirth in almost every culture. Only the most deprived and poverty-stricken resume work immediately. When there is time for any leisure at all in a society, it is generally given to the new mother, for it is recognized that the events in the first days and weeks after the birth can be as momentous as the birth itself.

The changes that take place after birth are extraordinary. On a purely physical level, in the process of recuperating from the strains of the labor and birth, the mother's body passes through rapid adjustments in her hormonal balance and in her blood supply. In addition to these physical changes, there are the complicated social and emotional changes that come with the transition from being an "expectant" parent to becoming a "real" parent. The entire family must adjust to the presence of the baby and acknowledge their own new relationship. This is not a simple matter. New babies take some getting used to—and so do new family roles.

The older couple is more likely to have thoroughly prepared itself mentally and emotionally for the new infant than the younger couple. The older mother's hormonal adjustments after the birth may be as variable and as difficult to cope with as those of the younger woman, but we found that the ability to cope was enhanced by having thought about those changes more beforehand, and also by simply being able to accept them in one's stride.

Since there is so much upheaval going on in the mother's body, in the family's roles, and in everybody's emotions, it is wise to keep the external changes to a minimum. That is why many families try to create a quiet nest for the early post partum weeks. They try to eliminate as many disturbances as possible. This may mean asking friends not to phone or visit, setting limits on the amount of time other family members can come over, and, in general, planning very carefully for a period of peace in which the new family can discover their own new lives slowly. As they get to know each other better, as the mother grows stronger and the baby becomes better adjusted to the conditions of the outside world, they can gradually resume a life that is more connected to things outside the home.

We talked at length with Alice, a woman who had a strong "nesting instinct." She had had a Caesarean section and so had more physical symptoms to recover from than most new mothers. She was very tired for the first few weeks and knew that she had to be very careful. She described her experience:

> We came home after two and a half days in the hospital. I could sleep for the first time here. I couldn't in the hospital. I was too excited at first, then too curious. People came in to check my blood pressure in the middle of the night. Then I had a roommate who watched TV most of the time, and we'd have maybe twenty visitors in a night. They were all people I loved, but I was *exhausted* and wanted to conserve my

strength for taking care of the baby. I was really very relieved to come home.

We decided to shut ourselves off. People got a little annoyed with us, but we decided we had to get to know ourselves as a threesome. I needed a lot of rest, but I think actually Alan was the most tired. He had been up with me throughout the labor, and he was the one who had to do all the practical things, like phone everybody, and get the house ready for us, and do the shopping.

We unplugged the phone and slept for the first day or so. The baby slept for four or five hours at a stretch then, and was real easy. He doesn't now that he's a month old, but he did then and we were able to recuperate.

Alan did all of the cooking and we had friends who brought us meals. They just left them at the door. Our childbirth education teacher suggested that. I was in bed pretty much all that first day and the next. Alan brought the baby to me and I nursed him in bed. Then I started to get up and around. By starting so gradually, we were able to deal with the physical exhaustion.

Alan was on a two-week vacation. I don't know how we could have done it otherwise. I guess you could get somebody else in to help, but it may be a drain emotionally to have someone else around. We were both just really relaxed, sleeping when the baby slept and being up together. In the third week, we all went to a friend's house for dinner, which worked out well, but I had to be careful not to get too tired. This week I went out alone for the first time. Alan was home and stayed with the baby while I just drove down to the shopping center. It was grand—I felt like a teenager, free to go off on my own like that. But I also thought of the baby the whole time. It felt strange being away from him. I'm still heavy and thick in the waist, and my breasts are full of milk for him. There's no way I can forget about him. He's just in my mind all the time, like he used to be in my body.

Alice was 34 when her son was born. She had waited many years to have her baby and did not feel in any rush to get out of the house. He was born in December, over Christmas vacation. She had been teaching school, but had resigned with the understanding that the school was interested in hiring her back the next year if she wanted to resume working. She was not sure what she would do about that, but neither was she worried about it. As she was getting more energetic and as the baby was getting easier to care for, she was starting projects around the house. Alan had arranged his schedule to be around the house as much as possible also. Even after a month, she felt as though she was still "inside the glow of the whole birth experience."

Not every woman is in a position to be as relaxed and comfortable as Alice in the early weeks after the baby is born. For "nesting-in" to work at home, a new mother must have people she loves and trusts to help her. She may be well enough to get out of bed on a limited basis, but she should not have to take over complete housekeeping and infant-care chores.

Alice was lucky to have Alan's devoted help. He was as involved with the newborn as she was. During the first two weeks, he did everything but breastfeed the infant. Both of them were comfortable with letting the housekeeping go while they spent their energy on looking after the baby and adjusting emotionally to new factors.

Another woman who tried to create the same situation found that even though her husband took off two weeks from work, she did not feel she really had a chance to be with him. He was busy with housekeeping and cooking and diaper-changing and visiting with friends who had come by. She felt they were never alone together. Then when he suddenly resumed work after the two weeks, he was away long hours and she was alone with no help. She wished that she had stayed in the hospital longer and hired someone else to take care of the house so that she and her husband could have had time to be together in peace and quiet.

Many families turn to the new mother's mother as the obvious person to help out in the post partum period. This is often a very happy solution for everyone. The new grandmother gets to know her new grandchild; the new mother receives the love and advice of her own mother; and the new father is relieved of some of the burdens of household management. For such a system to work, however, the generations must be comfortable with each other. Very young women may be happy to have their mothers take over because they are used to relying on them. Older women, however, may be ambivalent about the idea of returning to a state of being cared for by their mother after their years of growing independent. When it works well, the new intimacy across the generations can be one of the best parts of having a baby. Many women have told us how much closer they have grown to their own mothers during this period. If they share the same values, the mother can reassure the daughter about details of infant care and teach her little tricks of mothering. One daughter said, "I was afraid I would spoil the baby by picking it up too much, but Mom told me no, you can't spoil an infant, so I felt all right about doing what I wanted to do anyway." Another said:

> She sort of sets the way for me, saying it's okay to do this, it's okay if you leave him for a couple of hours, it's okay: "I'll take care of him so you can get out." She's a very aggressive woman and

isn't afraid of her own opinions, yet she is gentle. A couple of times she has wanted me to do something a certain way and I've just ignored it. I'm not afraid of her taking over, either. I thought I might be, but I'm enjoying her. It's not a threat. She says it's okay to let the baby cry sometimes, but I still have trouble with that.

Obviously, not all mother-daughter relationships are ideal. Sometimes the baby adds to the strain; sometimes it diminishes it. A woman named Helen said that she had always felt comfortable with her mother, but was shocked when the older woman asked, "Do you feel that we did something badly for you? Is that why you are doing things differently than we did them?" Helen found herself confused by these questions and by other remarks her mother made. By the time the baby was two weeks old, she and her husband had set limits on the amount of time they would spend with the two sets of grandparents. They felt that the older generation was making exhausting demands on them rather than helping things go more smoothly. Another woman, Lori, had the opposite experience. She had always known that she did not want to be like her own mother. It was her great fear throughout pregnancy. When the baby was finally born, she found that she could be more comfortable with her mother than ever before in her life:

> She's changed. She still gets obsessive about things and that brings out the same thing in me, which is what I don't like about myself, but the baby brings out positive things in her. She doesn't have the responsibility, so she doesn't have the guilt. She can just sort of let herself be a more giving person. She's a much more secure and happy person than she was when my sister and I were growing up.
> Having a baby has changed our relationship.

The things that used to drive me crazy about her bother me less because I found out I didn't need to be like her and I'm not like she was. Now our relationship is really good.

If the mother's mother or father's mother or any other relative can really help, they may be wonderful to have around. It seems particularly meaningful for the new parents to have family around them so that they can have a chance to explore their new status with those they love. For a new mother, this means receiving validation as a mother. However, families bring strong emotions and old patterns with them. These may be more negative than positive. One new mother described the arrival of her family after the baby's birth as "just fundamental chaos. We were all glad when they left." Sometimes families can be more burdensome than helpful.

Many families hire help for the post partum period. This generally takes the form of a cleaning person once or twice a week. Such an arrangement can take care of some of the most difficult practical problems of the period, as it frees the new parents from some of the demands of housework and cooking. They can have time to be together and to provide for the baby's needs, especially if the father is taking off from work for a week or two. If other family members come to visit, the new father and mother will not be under as much pressure to play host and hostess. If both parents are planning to resume work in the early months of the baby's life, it seems especially helpful to have a housekeeper who begins to work for the family before the baby is born and who can gradually assume care of the infant as the parents return to work.

Although having a housekeeper sounds like a rational and obvious solution to the housekeeping problems of the post partum period for anyone who can afford it, in practice it is not so simple. Particularly for older women, an added person in the house may seem like an intrusion. It may be more exhausting to have to deal with another person than to do the work. It also interferes with one's routine, which has probably been well established over a number of years.

Some families hire a baby nurse for the post partum period. This takes the strain of childcare off the new parents. For some, especially those who want to proceed with their lives with minimal interruption, this may be the ideal solution. Most new parents, however, want to assume the responsibilities of parenting themselves.

> At the last minute in the hospital I hired a baby nurse. This gave me the freedom when I got home to be out a great deal and it gave me the illusion my life hadn't changed—but it also made me feel I didn't have a baby. The love I had felt for her began to fade. I realized that even if I had the money for a "nanny" I wouldn't want to relinquish my relationship with my child.
>
> Since the nurse left, my child has begun to slowly recognize me and smile when I come in the room. I wouldn't trade those smiles for more freedom!

Many modern women, especially career women, feel ambivalent about the tradition of taking an extended time out after a baby is born. On the one hand, they can generally afford to take it easy without fear of severe economic consequences. Society at large will not suffer from their temporary absence. The husband can generally get along for two weeks or so while his wife recuperates in bed. But on the other hand, the woman herself is likely to feel that she must get up and go about her business as quickly as possible. This generation looks back with disdain on the generation of women who spent ten days in the hospital following childbirth. Now it is only five days, or two, or sometimes only a few hours before the new mother is discharged from the hospital. Certainly, a woman who has not been heavily medicated can be strong enough to go home very quickly after her baby is born. However, that does not mean that she has given up her "childbirth privilege." The early-release policies were begun because women complained that they could not rest in the hospital, or because a stay in the hospital was too expensive. They wanted to go home where there would be some peace and quiet, where they could be taken care of by their family and friends instead of by impersonal hospital staff. They wanted to be spared unnecessary hospital procedures and return to an environment where they felt comfortable. They wanted to stay with their husbands, their babies, and the rest of their families instead of lying alone in a strange bed in a strange room.

A woman who has come through the birth feeling healthy and strong still needs a period of "nesting-in." She has a lot to adjust to. So does her husband, her baby, and other members of the family. A quiet time at the very beginning can provide a secure basis for family relations.

Pregnancy was an exciting inner state that filled the woman with the idea of new life—a new life for herself as well as for the baby. When mother and child remain in intimate contact with each other for the first post partum months, this shared experience can be a happy and contented time for both. It is a gradual development from the union of pregnancy. When the separation occurs without sufficient emotional preparation by the mother, she may feel she has lost all that was valuable and alive within herself. She may feel depressed and empty. When the transition goes more smoothly, she can feel as though she is still within "the glow of the birth experience." The baby is in her arms instead of her womb, but is still excitingly present in her consciousness.

It may take quite a long time for a mother to get used to the new external reality of the child. In the early days or even weeks, it may be painful for a woman simply to be out of physical contact with her baby. After the emotional transition from inside to outside has been made, she will feel much more secure about leaving her baby for a while. Both mother and child gradually develop the ability to go for long periods of time without each other.

This is especially so for older parents. They should not be afraid to be overprotective of their children or over-involved in their children's lives and neglectful of their own personal activities. Ironically, it is the parents who don't have extended, intimate contact with their newborn who seem more likely to be over-involved later on. After the early weeks, a baby does not want to stay in a nest any more than a mother does. An eight-month-old needs to crawl around, to explore, to discover, just as the mother of an eight-month-old needs to play out her adult roles in society. Both mother and child gain strength and security in their new lives by emerging gradually.

Those women who are willing to suspend their other interests and activities for a few weeks and devote themselves to rest, recuperation, and acceptance of themselves as mothers have a smoother first month than those who are afraid of being isolated and struggle to do too much too soon.

A young, first-time mother may be afraid that she is going to lose touch with the world outside. The older mother seems less worried about losing touch with people and work. Her longer life experience tells her that little will happen in a few weeks or even a few months. Vacations take that long and people return from them with renewed strength and interest in their daily lives.

4
SPECIAL CONCERNS OF THE FIRST MONTHS

Breast Feeding

Almost all of the pregnant women with whom we have talked in the past few years have planned to breast feed their babies. This is especially true of women over 30, probably because they tend to be well-informed about health issues and have heard that breast milk is the best for the baby.

In the 1950's a breast-feeding mother was an oddity. This is no longer the case. Today, nurses, obstetricians, pediatricians, and midwives generally help women to nurse their babies and encourage them to continue doing it as long as possible. La Leche League, a support group for nursing mothers, provides advice and counseling for families who have questions or problems. Perhaps even more importantly, most new mothers are likely to have friends who have successfully nursed their babies, a circumstance that was simply not true even a few years ago. Some women are surprised to find that there is more support for breast feeding than for bottle feeding.

New childbirth practices have brought a positive influence to bear on successful breast feeding. When a new mother is alert and happy after the birth, she often wants to snuggle with her baby and bring it to her breast. Although her milk has not yet "come in,"—it probably will on the third or fourth day—her breasts are already producing *colostrum*, an almost clear, protein-rich fluid, which is one of the most important nutrients for the baby. Colostrum will pass the mother's immunities on to the baby, and it will allow the baby to gently adjust to the richer milk which the mother will offer a few days later. It is extremely important that the baby should not be deprived of colostrum. Frequently, nurses discourage mothers from nursing early, before the milk has appeared, and sometimes a mother will fear that the baby may not receive enough nourishment when she can only give a few drops of this clear fluid from her breasts. It is important to bear in mind that nature has provided a very safe food for the baby and that early sucking will stimulate the milk flow. Also, this initial exploratory encounter seems to facilitate the establishment of a good nursing relationship.

Every once in a while we still hear about a woman who did not have a chance to nurse her baby in the first hour after its birth. Sometimes this is unavoidable. A mother who has had a Caesarean section cannot suckle her baby while she is being stitched, not only because the infant might get in the way of the doctor's work, but also because the sucking causes contractions of the uterus, which would create problems with the stitching. Now that Caesareans are sometimes performed with a local anesthetic, the new mother may want to take her baby in her arms immediately and may be disappointed if she cannot. But if she has made visual contact with the baby, she should have no trouble nursing it as soon as this is possible. If the baby must be taken to another area for an extra examination or for special treatment, this separation may be very difficult for the mother, especially if she is wide awake and excited. But she, too, will be able to establish her nursing relationship later on. It will go most easily if both she and the baby are alert and relaxed when they are reunited.

Some hospitals still have a policy of separating the baby from the mother for twelve or more hours after the birth in order to have a pediatrician check the baby. This routine separation makes it hard for the mother to establish a breast-feeding schedule from the very beginning. Some hospitals still give sugar water to babies in the nursery, instead of letting the mother supply the beneficial colostrum. The rationale for the sugar water seems to be that possible difficulties in swallowing may be determined more easily with the intake of sugar water than colostrum.

While we agree that it is important that the baby be checked carefully soon after birth, we feel this could be easily done in a family-oriented way, by not separating the baby from its parents while it is being observed.

Breast feeding, like lovemaking, is most enjoyable when it evolves gradually out of intimacy and sensuality. It is less successful when forced or when performed from a sense of duty. Breast feeding involves "foreplay" which stimulates the interest of the infant and helps the mother's nipples grow erect. This foreplay often consists of the mother's cooing and cuddling and brushing her nipple across the baby's cheek. The baby's lips touch the mother's breast, it looks up into the mother's eyes, and pats its mother's skin with its tiny fingers. In the early hours after birth, it is more important that this loving relationship get started than that the baby get milk, for love provides a very important form of nourishment and assures a strong, caring relationship.

Many American women are sensitive about exposing their breasts. They certainly do not want to be touched there by strangers, and the baby may feel like a stranger to them at first. When the first encounter occurs immediately after the birth, the connection is more clear. The mother can then move most comfortably from holding, looking at, and touching the baby to nursing it. Nothing need be forced. The baby was not brought to her just to be nursed; it was placed in her arms to be encountered, to be loved. The nursing can flow naturally from this.

The decision to use a bottle can be a valid and sensible one. Most formulas provide excellent nutrition, and other caretakers can provide the same feeding situation as the mother. The baby needs the loving and cuddling of its mother, but this can be provided during bottle feedings and at other times. The milk from the breasts is only one small part of the interaction, and probably the part that can most easily be replaced. There is no substitute for love.

We are strongly in favor of breast feeding, but only when it is a happy experience for both the mother and child. It is true that the sucking action of the baby helps the uterus contract to its non-pregnant size. It is also true that breast milk provides immunity to some diseases, and that breast feeding is the most natural continuation of the close pregnancy relationship. But these advantages do not overcome all other considerations. For example, some women do not want to be bound by a physical relationship to their child. Others are embarrassed to expose their breasts. Some simply do not enjoy breast feeding or feel sure they will not enjoy it. Such women should be allowed to respect their own feelings and to choose the reasonable alternative of bottle feeding.

We are not worried about the families who choose to bottle feed and are sure of their decision. We are concerned, however, for women whose decision to nurse was made during pregnancy but who are unable to establish a comfortable breast-feeding relationship in the post partum period. When such women resort to the bottle, they feel that they are going against their original intentions and that, in this sense, they have failed. They may need help in understanding what has happened.

Sometimes a woman will say she wants to breast feed because it seems the thing to do, even though she really does not want to do it. She may be relieved if it "doesn't work." Then she will be able to stay: "I tried to do what was best but I couldn't."

In our experience, the situation is rarely that simple. Nurses, friends, and family cannot tell that the woman didn't really mean it when she said she wanted to breast feed. They will try to give well-intentioned advice which may increase the new mother's unspoken conflict between her desire to bottle feed and her feeling that she *ought* to nurse. As her feeling of guilt increases, she will become increasingly uncomfortable, both with herself and with the baby. This is obviously not a good situation for any member of the family.

The two most common explanations given by new mothers who try but fail to breast feed their babies are that the baby "didn't want to" (often experienced by the mother as a rejection), and that they don't have enough milk.

Perhaps there are some babies who do not want to nurse at the breast. Generally, however, this remark indicates a problem with the entire mother-infant relationship, rather than simply a problem with breast feeding. If breast feeding adds tension to the mother-infant relationship, it should certainly be abandoned in favor of finding ways to make that relationship more comfortable. A woman who is ambivalent about breast feeding may benefit from direction and help, but for some women encouragement just increases the sense of failure.

> I tried putting honey on my nipples and feeding her a taste of breast milk on a spoon. The public health nurse came to our house to help me out. I joined a new mothers group at the hospital in

which all the mothers were nursing. But nothing worked. She would scream and I would give her warm water, and finally I was sneaking formula and feeling guilty. I was getting more and more tense and upset. I was embarrassed and ashamed and guilty and upset. Finally my husband suggested that the baby was crying because I was upset. He said *he* would be more comfortable if I stopped trying because I was getting more hysterical each day. After that I started giving her the formula regularly and things calmed down a lot. I could even relax and let her nurse a couple of times a day. She'd often do it for five minutes or so and once suckled a long time, about twenty minutes. In a sense I guess I did let her nurse for the first five months, but I don't really think of it that way. I wasn't using the breast for nourishment, and my milk was pretty much gone by the time she was six months old.

It was a terrible time for me at first. Fortunately, my husband was wise and really helped me out by trying to understand what would be best for me. Everybody else made me feel guilty, but he didn't. And my mother was a big help. I talked to her on the telephone a lot during that time, even though we live so far apart. She is a nurse, but she had had trouble breast feeding also. She said all three of us fussed and wouldn't do it, just like my baby.

Breast feeding can be handled in many different ways. The woman quoted above did use the breast, but not for the major source of nourishment. The formula was the basis, while the breast was supplemental to her baby's feeding schedule. Other women do the opposite. They rely on the breast for basic nourishment in the early months and occasionally give a bottle as a supplement. Many women introduce an occasional or even a daily bottle quite soon after nursing is established because they want to be able to leave the baby with someone else. Frequently, this is for the benefit of the husband, who wants an intimate relationship with the child and feels that feeding will help establish the kind of nurturing warmth that he wants to experience. In other cases, the bottle is used by a babysitter or grandmother while the parents are away.

Sometimes the supplementary bottles contain breast milk rather than formula. Many mothers want to be sure their babies have their milk, so they express it into a bottle and refrigerate it for later use.

Even babies who are exclusively on the breast are fed in different ways. Some mothers believe the breast should always be available. They carry the baby close to their bodies in a sling and sleep with it at their sides. The baby rapidly becomes adroit at finding the nipple when she or he wants it. Other mothers generally keep the nipple away from the baby, but give it on demand. Whenever the baby cries, the mother picks it up and nurses it. Some other mothers rely on a schedule to know when to feed the baby. They let it nurse at regular times of the day and night and for pre-determined periods of time. While this is efficient for the mother, it may not be a realistic method of taking care of an infant's changing needs during a period of rapid growth.

Women often experience anxieties related to breast feeding. Because they cannot tell how much the baby has taken, they wonder whether or not it has eaten enough. Whenever the baby cries, they are likely to think that it is hungry or to worry that their milk is inadequate. Some mothers have discovered that the breast is not the answer to all of the baby's problems. They comfort it through holding and rocking instead of always at the breast. An older baby may want to be played with or distracted rather than fed when it is uncomfortable.

Mothers should be aware that while babies develop a relationship to the breast which is partially based on the need for comfort and love, their need for nourishment takes up a great deal of time.

> I expected it to be different. I thought she should go a couple of hours between nursing, but my mother would say, "She's hungry." So I'd nurse her. She eats eight to twelve times a day. I didn't know it would be like that.

With the baby spending so much time at the breast, the mother must come to terms with her own feelings about being available for so much feeding. She must relax and sit comfortably while the baby eats. She may also feel that she must give the baby her total attention the entire time. Women remark that they feel guilty about wanting to read or perform some other activity while breast feeding. They want to be all-giving and all-patient, but sometimes they admit to having had enough of it. This seems to be increasingly the case as the baby gets older. What was an exciting event at three weeks can become a bit boring by five months. Fortunately, the baby is also getting ready to move on to other things. It wants to eat some solid foods. It wants to spend more time looking around and playing and less time being cuddled and suckled. An older baby may flirt and play and tease more than it suckles. These are wonderful and delightful interactions, but sometimes the mother has other things to do. Women who become skilled at "reading" their child's needs learn how to resolve this dilemma. They set aside a few quiet hours during the day to nurse the baby in peace and quiet. Then they let the other meals include some solid foods, with the confidence that if the baby is playing more than it is drinking, it is more playful than hungry. They can carry the baby in a body strap or place it in an infant seat while they go about their business, playing with the baby and taking care of chores at the same time.

Many women continue to breast feed only until the baby is about six months old. Others continue through the first year or until the baby can hold a cup. Some allow the child to take comfort from the breast as long as it wants.

Some women feel comforted by breast feeding. For others, while the intimacy of a quiet period of breast feeding is very wonderful, the tugs of a nine-month-old trying to lift a blouse may simply be annoying. Some women, therefore, want to stop breast feeding before the baby becomes overly willful or before its teeth come in.

There are many different philosophies about when to introduce solid foods. A lot depends on the maturity of the baby's digestive tract and its particular caloric needs. Most mothers introduce foods by trial and error, while following the advice of the baby's pediatrician. It is important for the mother and the doctor to have similar ideas about how food should be handled. A mother who lacks faith in her own breast milk may have trouble being comfortable with her doctor's suggestion that she rely exclusively on nursing for a number of months. Conversely, a woman who does not trust solid foods and who wants to provide for the baby's needs from her own body for as long as possible will be distrustful of her doctor's suggestions about introducing solid foods early. The parents should choose a doctor carefully. It is important that they trust his advice and that they feel free to question him about any and all issues.

Some women go through a difficult period during which they think that their milk is drying up. The milk may occasionally dry up when the mother is under a great deal of stress. Often babies wean themselves; they simply decide for some reason of their own that they have had enough of the mother's milk and want to enter their next phase. When women start their babies on solids, when they go back to work, or when anything traumatic occurs, the milk supply can be affected. It may be hard for a woman who would like to go on nursing to find that for some reason the baby is no longer very interested in her milk. She may experience it as a kind of rejection of herself. Often advice from a pediatrician or someone from La Leche League or the Nursing Mothers' Council will be enough to assure the mother that she can continue. She may have to take life easy for two or three days and just cuddle up with the baby in bed until it resumes nursing on its own. This usually works beautifully in reestablishing the milk supply. However, some women really do not want to spend three days in bed with the baby. They may feel that their milk had begun to run out because they themselves were getting tired of breast feeding. It may be harder to admit that one simply doesn't want to continue breast feeding than to say: "My milk has dried up." It means giving up a little more of the image of being a perfect parent. But it may be the most realistic solution for a woman who wants her body to return to normal as quickly as possible.

The question of when to wean the baby is a complex one which involves both the needs of the baby and the needs of the mother. Even when the woman rationally decides that it is time to wean, the process may still be unexpectedly difficult because of a sense of loss of the early mother-infant intimacy. Weaning symbolizes a major step towards the growing child's eventual independence. This makes it a bittersweet time.

Because we have been talking about problems and not successes, it may seem as though breast feeding is a very delicate matter. In fact, however, most women find that it is quite simple, even during periods of stress or change.

Some women say: "What should I do when I go

back to work?" Although we have known many women who weaned their babies before returning to work, we have also known many who continued to breast feed even while working full time. In such cases, while not the sole means of nourishment, breast feeding continues to be enjoyed for the special intimacy of the situation. A working mother shared her feelings with us:

> He obviously knows the difference between me and the housekeeper, but I wonder if he knows who's the Mommy. She's important to his family constellation. He greets her with great joy. On weekends we sometimes wonder if he misses her. She has all day to play with him.
> He has this wonderful all-day relationship with her. I do try to be around when he goes to bed and when he gets up, but sometimes I wonder who's the more important to him. But then I remember that I am the Mommy. I am the one who nurses him. That is our special bond.

Women who are well into breast feeding and have been doing it for several months speak in glowing terms about the experience. They love the special feeling, the intimacy connected to it. The quiet times of nursing in the middle of the night or early in the morning become special moments of peace and joy. Alone with the baby, free from distractions, the nursing mother can become aware of her profound relationship to the baby in a way that she cannot in the midst of a busy day.

> Last night, as I was nursing our ten-week-old, she stopped sucking and stared at me intently for a minute. As we gazed into each other's eyes, she smiled and cooed with pleasure, and I was overwhelmed with the strength of the bond that

has formed between us. The creation of a new life is a miracle and a glory.

These are very special moments and will always stand out in a woman's memories of early mothering. There are few differences between women who are over 30 and those who are 25 in relation to breast feeding. The milk supply does not seem to be affected by age, as far as we now know. The worries and joys of breast feeding seem to vary with the individual rather than with age.

Sex

We have written an entire book, *Making Love During Pregnancy,* to discuss the problems and pleasures in sex experienced by couples during pregnancy and the post partum period. We will not go into detail here, but we would like to mention some of the major changes that generally occur. They can be disturbing to couples who do not anticipate them.

It is hard to remember that until she has recovered from childbirth, and to some extent as long as she is nursing, a woman's body and her sexual responsiveness are influenced by her involvement in reproduction. The physiological changes that occur during pregnancy, birth, and the post partum period manifest themselves in the sex organs and inevitably create changes in sexual functioning. A woman's sexual parts are actually physically different during and immediately after pregnancy than they were before she became pregnant, and this has a profound effect—emotional as well as physical—on sex. We can use the breasts to illustrate the nature of the changes that occur.

Early in pregnancy, the breasts grow sensitive and even painful to the touch. Later they become enlarged, and often more susceptible to erotic stimulus than they had been previously. Finally, after the baby is born, they miraculously provide the baby with all the food it needs. As we described in the last section, breast feeding can be an intimate and rewarding experience for both the mother and the infant.

The very intensity of the nursing relationship can carry with it certain sexual problems. For a few women, the baby's sucking is quite erotic. This can be disturbing for the woman who feels that sexual arousal is not an appropriate response under the circumstances. Generally, the feelings are sensual rather than truly sexual, but every once in a while a woman will have an orgasm while breast feeding her baby.

Breasts are generally thought of as erotic in our culture. Indeed, stimulation of the breasts can cause sexual arousal even when it is produced by an infant rather than by a lover. This confusion between the erotic and the maternal can be disconcerting, and it may result in the feeling—on the part of both men and women—that it is inappropriate to use the breasts, which now seem to belong to the baby, in sex play.

The breasts also pose some practical problems for sex during the post partum period. Because of the connection between the erotic and the maternal systems, sexual arousal often releases the flow of milk. Some women either have to express the extra milk from their breasts before lovemaking or expect to get wet. This inconvenience is more troubling to some couples than to others A few rather enjoy it; some women do not experience it at all.

Of course, the sexual changes that occur in the childbearing year manifest themselves in other areas besides the breasts. The breasts are tied in with the larger system of change. Just as the enlargement of the breasts is triggered by the pregnancy, and their ability to lactate by the birth, so too the use of the breasts in nursing can cause changes in the vagina and the uterus. Initially the baby's sucking stimulates hormones that produce contractions of the uterus and speed its return to health and normalcy. As breast feeding goes on, it functions to suppress ovulation. This means that a woman is less likely to get pregnant again and displace the infant who still relies on her body for survival. It also means that her sexual hormones are suppressed.

A woman who is breast feeding sometimes finds that she is not as sexually responsive as usual. There are many reasons for this. She is often tired from lack of sleep, and she may be run down from the heavy routine of childcare. She may also feel more closely linked with her infant than with her husband, and may not want to become involved in a sexual encounter with an adult. But underlying all these other factors, there is also a hormonal situation that tends to make a woman unresponsive. This may be particularly difficult for a husband to understand. He is likely to feel rejected and jealous.

All of the changes that occur in a woman's body during the childbearing year are associated with giving birth to and nurturing the baby. Unfortunately, when couples are acutely aware of themselves as mothers and fathers, they sometimes feel that they should not be enjoying sex together. It is often difficult to accept the parallels between the sexual response cycle and the entire progress of the childbearing year. In both cases, the woman starts off at her usual base point, then progresses through changes in her hormonal balance and in her blood supply, particularly in the vaginal area. Under both circumstances, she experiences vaginal lubrication. Finally, at the culminating point of both experiences, rhythmic contractions of the uterus, vagina, and entire perineal area occur.

Obviously, birth is far more complicated and dramatic than orgasm, but the two events have a great deal in common, both physiologically and psychologically. They both are accompanied by a sense of opening up and of accepting a strong love relationship. In both cases, the woman's body expands to permit the passage of the loved one into her vagina. Then, in both cases, the woman's body passes into a phase of lowered estrogen. Her vagina changes, lubricates less, and has thinner, drier walls. Although she may be capable of starting the cycle of arousal again, it will take her longer.

Although it may be thought of as a wonderful and exciting thing that the baby emerges from its mother's body through a process that is related to the way that it began, it may also be scary. Most men are thrilled and excited to watch the birth of their baby, but some become quite disturbed by the changes they witness in the vagina. It is hard to believe that a body can be so elastic that it can accommodate the passage of a baby, and yet return to a size that is appropriate for lovemaking. Any fears that do get stirred up are not easy to reconcile, for a woman *is* different after childbirth.

The post partum period is a time of adjustment. The baby requires so much love and attention that other members of the family often feel there is no love left over for them. Both parents are likely to be tired from lack of sleep. The mother's perineum is sore and her breasts are leaky. The first attempt at lovemaking is often disappointing or even disastrous. The woman's vagina may be tight and dry. The man is afraid of hurting her. He may be amazed to find himself impotent. After a bad first experience, it may be hard to try again.

Mature couples who have been together a long time have a distinct advantage over younger, less experienced couples. They are more likely to have been through other periods of sexual difficulty in their relationship and to know that there is a normal ebb and flow of desire even when the strains of childbearing do not intervene. They also know that a period of exciting, wonderful lovemaking can come even after a rather long stretch of disinterest. It may be a bit easier for them to be relaxed and loving together and to be more patient about awaiting the return of their more engrossing erotic encounters.

The Post Partum Blues

The post partum blues are not a single phenomenon with a single cause. The term is a catch-all used to cover all the bad feelings that a mother may have in the first days, weeks, or months after a baby is born.

Some women find themselves crying for no apparent reason as they pack their bags to leave the hospital on the third day after the birth. Others drag themselves through months of feeling half-alive. Approximately 4000 American women require hospitalization each year for serious mental illness that occurs during the year after a baby's birth. Such severe cases sometimes follow the birth of a first child, but they seem more likely to occur after a third child with the accumulated stress of the childbearing year and the already heavy demands on the woman's emotions and energy.

Such periods of depression may take place in the first five post partum days, in the first four post partum weeks, or not until the second post partum month or even later. Since there are so many different kinds of post partum depression, it is inevitable that there should be many different causes as well. It is probably rare for any woman to be depressed for only one reason. Every case of the blues could probably supply enough causes to fill the pages of a novel. Each woman's situation is unique, and the reasons for her reaction are probably linked to her entire life experience. Nevertheless, there are certain shared factors. If we can clarify some of the contributing causes, we may be able to create an environment that will minimize the effects of the blues.

THE PHYSIOLOGICAL COMPONENT

Pregnancy, childbirth, and nursing all entail profound biochemical upheavals. They involve many of the body systems, but most particularly they involve changes in such hormones as estrogen and in steroids which are known to affect moods. Even women who do not feel depressed after the birth may be aware of distinct changes occurring within their bodies. For women who found the changes of pregnancy euphoric, the changes of the post partum period are likely to be depressing, on a purely physical level. Some women, however, have the opposite experience.

> My old hormones are back, and that has given me a very big lift. When I got pregnant, I became a totally different person. The return happened last week (two and a half weeks post partum). I could literally feel it. In fact, I broke out in pimples. It was like going through adolescence or something. I feel like being with people again. I feel like doing things. I just feel better. I feel great!

While this woman's experience may be extreme, it does indicate the extent to which women feel their bodies changing. It is very important for new mothers to pay special attention to their diet and to consider the possible need for dietary supplements under their health professional's supervision throughout the post partum period. Breast feeding also makes special demands on a woman's body and requires adequate nutrition to compensate for calories and nutrients consumed by the baby. By keeping up her health and strength, she may be more likely to avoid depression.

The physiological changes surrounding birth contribute to many aspects of the blues. However, there are undoubtedly social and emotional factors at work as well. They go beyond the physiological changes. The most distinct proof is that parents who adopt children may also be subject to depression soon after they receive a child.

The mind and the body interact far too subtly for a simple solution to such a complex problem. We must assume that a physiological component is at work, but that it interacts with the normal and exceptional stresses of the period as well as with the underlying psychology of the person involved.

ROUTINE STRESS

Labor and birth are both physically and emotionally exhausting. When they are experienced as a great high, the period afterwards may be quite a letdown, simply because it is not as dramatic. When labor and birth are not experienced as a great high, the new parents may become obsessed with their disappointment. Even a good birth cannot guarantee a happy post partum period, but we believe that a smooth and happy birth with continual parent-infant contact does eliminate or minimize many of the feelings of shock or sorrow or abandonment that can occur in the early days.

We have frequently found that the prepared and older mother has far fewer difficulties of adjustment, mainly because she and her husband prepared longer and better for this period of change.

There are many stories of tears and hurt feelings that seem to have resulted from unfortunate but avoidable circumstances. For example, women often describe bursting into tears when a nurse is gruff or critical. They talk about the despair they feel when they aren't allowed to hold their baby and the loneliness that comes when, after being the center of attention for several hours, they are wheeled to their hospital room while their husbands go to the nursery with the baby. One woman told us that, though she couldn't understand why, she found herself sobbing uncontrollably when she was told it was time to leave the hospital. Another burst into tears when she was told she would have to have a roommate and her husband wouldn't be allowed to sleep with her in the hospital.

These incidents may sound trivial to those of us who have not had a baby, and perhaps they would seem so to the women who experienced them under other conditions. But these intense responses to minor details are characteristic of the fragility of women's emotions after birth. It is not a time in which to be objectively distanced from the situation. It is a time of overwhelming involvement with every detail. The woman's body has been wrenched open; both it and her psyche are still incredibly vulnerable. If she overreacts to every little slight, it may be because of her awareness of the discrepancy between her profound experience and the routine existence of others around her.

A woman needs to feel secure and trusting in the hours and days around birth. When anyone or anything makes her feel insecure, the total vulnerability of her situation may rush in on her. She needs to be taken care of and to be loved. She has good reason to panic if she feels neglected or unloved. The task in front of her is a vast one. She must assume responsibility for the life of another human being. At the same time she is feeling weak and tender. She needs to feel secure about the process of gradually discovering her own way of caring for her infant and interacting with her family.

Even though we have just written a section on "nesting-in," and have stressed its importance, the fact is that most families cannot achieve that ideal. Some babies sleep a great deal and let the mother rest, but others cry almost continuously. Some husbands will cook and clean house and cuddle their wives to make them feel loved and important, but others make extraordinary demands to be cared for themselves. Some families quietly tiptoe in to leave a pot roast on the back burner, but others sit at the foot of the new mother's bed and tell her disapproving stories about other people's babies, making her exhausted and on edge. And last but not least, some women are content to take a few weeks for quiet recuperation, but others have a need to get out and have contact with people, to stay in touch with the world about them. They would rather risk exhaustion than isolation.

> To me, post partum depression is explainable. If a woman doesn't have supporting friends and husband, my God, I'd be depressed. I got to the point of wanting to take the phone off the hook, I got so many calls, but it made such a difference. I'm not going to be isolated.

This woman felt the ambiguity of needing friends and at the same time longing for the phone to keep quiet and give her a rest.

Another woman was pushed over her limit by well-intentioned family and friends. Her parents, her husband's parents, and her sister came to stay for lengthy periods. In addition, the couple had many friends and neighbors who constantly stopped by to admire the baby.

> It was just too much and I was really exhausted. If and when we have another child, I won't do that ever again, because I was just falling apart

a lot, getting hysterical and crying just because I was so tired. I couldn't function.

The routine stress of birth goes beyond the few days that would be needed to recuperate if there were not a child to be cared for. Even apart from the rigors of childbirth, caring for a newborn can be exceedingly stressful. Many new parents feel anxious about whether or not they will be able to fulfill the needs of a helpless, dependent human being. At the same time, they are likely to experience overwhelming fatigue from loss of sleep and intense frustration at listening to the baby cry and not being able to do anything about it.

Even when the new parents are patient and content to devote themselves to their infant's care for the first few weeks, they may feel their fatigue and their frustration mounting. As the weeks go by, the newness of the situation fades. Friends and family stop calling and visiting, for it is no longer a special event. The father resumes his full working schedule, which means that he has less energy to devote to the family and more reason to want an undisturbed night of sleep. The mother may realize that she is not getting out of the house as much as she had assumed she would. While she had had a great deal of support, increasingly she may feel on her own.

Even though I'd been around babies a lot and newborns too, and both Ken and I have always been great with kids, it has been hard. I thought I'd just jump in there and that it would be a snap, but I have really been scared a lot of the time.
    One day when the baby was about ten days old, Ken had to leave in the afternoon and he didn't get home until two a.m. It was horrible. The baby cried all night, just off and on all night long. When Ken finally came home I was just

> like a puddle sitting here just wringing wet and holding the baby and we were both crying. It was horrible, really horrible. I had always thought I was an older mother and could handle all those difficult things I had heard about, but that time things were quite bad. Luckily that was the only time.

Descriptions of desperate situations like this are not unusual in the early post partum months. They seem to involve a combination of fatigue, frustration, and fear. The remarkable thing is that they tend to go hand in hand with the pleasure and contentment that women take in having the child and with their love for the child itself. When women talk about despair, about loneliness, about the unrelenting demands the baby makes upon them, and about their resentment at not being free to do what they want to do when they want to do it, they still come back to their feelings of love for the baby and their conscientious desire to do what is best.

The new restrictions imposed by the presence of the baby contribute to the stress of the post partum period. No move is ever completely free. If the parent who is the primary caretaker (almost always the mother) is not going to be with the baby herself, then she must make sure that someone else is there.

> At four months, I still get overwhelmingly tired. I still get very frustrated that I don't get time to do other things, not necessarily creative things; just *other*. It's just him all the time and housework, which I hate, but wind up doing constantly. The conflicts are just there.

Sometimes these feelings are so deep that nothing seems to relieve them. A woman may feel them even when she has the help of a considerate husband, a visiting mother, and a part-time babysitter:

Even with my mom here getting up in the night and Ed getting up in the night, I still found I just couldn't catch up on sleep. It was just being with the baby and not being with an adult and not getting out. She kept me in the house all day and I felt that I was being stifled.

Life at home with a baby is radically different from the life of most thirty-year-old, childless people. Old patterns of sleeping, eating, working, and playing are all disrupted. Over and over again new parents remark in amazement that taking care of an infant is the hardest job they have ever done. It consumes more time and energy than anyone can possibly anticipate. This may be as true for a woman in her thirties as for one in her twenties. A thirty-seven-year-old woman remarked:

I now have a respect for mothers that I never had before. I was always a little contemptuous of them and didn't understand why you couldn't easily combine work and a career with being a parent. I felt I *knew* what hard work was. After all, didn't I work seven days a week and sometimes twelve hours a day at that? What a shock to find it was *nothing* compared to the work of mothering. I tried to describe it to someone who had no children, and said it was a little like what the "Burma March" must have been like. The erosive quality of the tiredness is unlike anything I've ever known. Knowing that I *must* answer to another person's needs is totally exhausting.

With so much stress inherent in the months after the birth of a baby, the new parents need all the help and support they can get. Unfortunately, our society is no longer very sensitive to the needs of parents. Childcare has become an exceedingly low-prestige activity. A woman who chooses to stay home to take care of her baby finds she is apologizing that she is "just" a housewife. Many modern women have an intense fear of falling into the "housewife syndrome." They worry that their lives will change for the worse, that they will become guilt-ridden and dull. These fears can lead to a frantic attempt to stay active in the world, an attempt that may lead to increased stress and fatigue.

But there are now very good signs that post-natal groups are forming. There are self-help groups and groups led by professionals. There are also "hotlines" and "warmlines" that parents can call when difficulties arise. Early childhood development classes are being formed all over the country and La Leche League, an organization of dedicated women who help other women with breast feeding problems, has always been a firm supporter of new parents of all ages.

Having a baby necessitates change, changes in lifestyle, changes in thinking, and changes in relating to those around us. All of these changes may be challenging, exhilarating and exciting, but they may also cause severe stress.

It is common for a family to move before or after a baby is born. There will be new needs for space, but it is also often a symbolic move, to a "better" neighborhood, perhaps where the schools are better, to the suburbs, to the country, to a house with a better yard, to an apartment building with a playground. The rationales are many, but the underlying motive seems to be a desire to reflect the overwhelming internal changes inherent in becoming a parent by making a concomitant set of external changes.

Many of the stresses associated with taking care of an infant cannot be avoided; a certain number of them, however, could be. Since change generally creates a certain amount of stress, it is probably best to let the baby be the only significant change for the year, putting off other changes to a time when child-care has become easier and more of a routine and the baby can adjust more easily to new measures.

THE PSYCHOLOGICAL COMPONENT

There is no one kind of personality that will predictably become depressed in the post partum period. The psychological factors at work are complex and interact with physiological changes and with social stresses in ways that are unique for individual families. There are several psychological theories that try to explain the "baby blues." Each one probably holds true for certain individuals, but no one theory is likely to apply to everyone who feels disturbingly depressed after a baby is born.

We have found that there are far fewer depressions among women who prepared for childbirth. We saw from our talks with the older parents that women who wait to have a baby often have no post partum depression, simply because they have greater self-control and understanding and less resentment at having their lives altered so overwhelmingly.

However, a few of the theories that attempt to explain the factors that may trigger off feelings of depression are worth looking at.

Underlying Personality Problems

Some of the women who experience problems after the birth of a child were psychologically unstable to begin with. Any psychological difficulty can become more extreme under stress. All of us have limits to our emotional endurance just as we have limits to our physical endurance. The birth of a baby—and even the pregnancy itself—can contribute to either a physical or mental weakening or even a breakdown although it may also help a woman feel stronger and better about herself.

It is hard to predict whether a given individual will feel better or worse after the baby is born. Sometimes women who feel anxious during pregnancy feel much better after they are able to hold and care for the baby. Conversely, a certain number of women who are euphoric during pregnancy and can't wait to have the baby are unable to cope with the period after the birth. Having a baby is not a solution to a woman's emotional problems; neither is it necessarily the cause of her emotional problems. But it is such an overwhelming event that it may very well exacerbate whatever emotional difficulties a person may have.

Identity Crisis

Contemporary psychologists often refer to the early stages of parenthood as a period of crisis. According to this way of thinking, a person in crisis is in the midst of a profound transformation and reevaluation of his or her identity. When an identity transformation is taking place, the individual will experience his or her whole life as being in flux. The solidity of one's sense of self may seem to be shattered while a new structure is in the process of being created. Since an entirely new set of adjustments may be necessary to deal with the changed realities in the life of a person who is undergoing such a transformation, it is obvious that dealing with such crises produces significant growth and development. It is quite unrealistic to fight such changes. The mature person will greet them with delight and will work on becoming a new, different, and perhaps even happier individual. The younger parent may have more difficulties, but will eventually also find her new self.

During any crisis there is likely to be a revival of conflicts from the past. Around the time of pregnancy, men and women typically remember feelings from their own infancy, especially feelings connected to their own parents. It has been our repeated experience (and that of many others) that regression can take place during any illness and particularly during a hospital stay. The atavistic fear of the "medicine man" causes additional fears and anxieties. In the case of parents, their state of vulnerability around the time of the birth can bring about the loss of self-assertion and even regression to feelings of childish helplessness. Such emotions at the same time cause doctors and nurses almost unconsciously to play up to the role which has been placed on them. The great advantage here for older parents is that they are much more able to reintegrate their egos on a more mature level, whereas a very young parent may find this an almost overwhelming task.

A woman who has invested too much of her ego in identifying with the fetus is likely to have an unrealistic perception of a mother's ability to protect her infant after it is born. She may want to be able to provide everything, as she did in pregnancy. She wants to be a perfect mother, which means caring perfectly for the baby, loving it totally and unambivalently, and never letting it cry or be alone. In practice, this is impossible. Babies cry and sometimes they cannot be comforted. The baby and the mother are not one blissful madonna-and-child unit *all* the time. When the mother finds herself getting angry or feeling neglected, she will be unable to deal with her feelings. She is likely to feel betrayed and abandoned by everyone—and especially by that perfect mother who was supposed to take care of the helpless little baby. She gets angry at the doctors, the nurses, her husband, the baby, and at society in general. The anger is likely to be directed at anyone and everyone who was supposed to take care of her and didn't.

It may take a while for a new mother who has over-identified with the baby to adjust to the reality of her situation and to discover that she can satisfy the daily needs of her newborn. She may never be able to fill the deeper, more pressing emptiness of the infant part of herself. She may be a person who feels unloved and who needs a great deal of nurturing and mothering. It may be hard to admit that she, the mother, should have such needs or that she is worthy of anyone else's love.

Identification with the fetus can manifest itself as a symptom of the regression which is so often characteristic of the childbearing period. It is generally, however, a very happy and positive part of the experience. It is wonderful that mothers and fathers feel deeply linked to their own infants. This basic identification is at the heart of parental emotions of empathy and love. Parents know that their children are a part of themselves. The bonds are real. Healthy parents use this link to help in their ability to care for the baby. Only occasionally does a parent lose track of the real situation and expect the baby to satisfy his or her own needs directly.

Because mother and infant are linked in such a profound symbiotic bond, it is easy for the mother to experience herself as the other half. The mother may think she is the infant; similarly, the child, who has never been successfully separated on an emotional level from its mother, can over-identify with its mother. To some extent, this is a positive development when a woman becomes a mother herself. Once she feels her deep identification with her own mother inside herself, she may feel secure in her own role as mother. She has incorporated a positive model and knows that it is good to be a parent.

Sometimes a woman feels threatened not only by the possibility of becoming *like* her own mother, but actually of *becoming* her own mother. It is a very real fear for those women who have never felt secure in their individuality or who know their own mothers to be women with whom they do not want to identify.

In speaking to older mothers, it seemed to us that

they were more secure and unthreatened in their image of themselves as a mother. Younger women may have a harder task because they are afraid of displacing their own mothers (who may still be of childbearing age), and because they are unready to accept the idea of being mothers themselves. A woman of any age who has an unrealistic idea of what a "good" mother should be may have trouble accepting her own fallibility in the post partum period. She may get depressed because she feels so inadequate.

Loss As a Cause of Depression

At any stage in life, depression can result from loss. If we are to look for losses that may explain post partum blues, they are not hard to find. Most conspicuously, the woman's former way of life has been lost. Youth, freedom, the carefree life—all these things seem to be gone forever. Sometimes it is almost impossible for a woman who is depressed to go beyond her subjective feeling of loss, and it is even more difficult to realize that with the loss of one kind of freedom, she is gaining exciting new experiences which are going to last a very long time.

Many a woman has cried for the person she used to be: the girl who played so naively with dolls, the teenager who danced until dawn, the young woman who was so proud of her paycheck, the wife who always kept the house spotless and had every meal ready on time. All of these former selves may seem to have been lost when a woman confronts the reality of mothering.

Theodore Reik adds another loss to this already formidable list. He has remarked that women get depressed in the post partum period because they have lost the pregnancy and the fetus. A woman who has a baby before she is "ready" will be more likely to experience a sense of loss.

Accepting Change

Theories of post partum depression indicate the importance of minimizing external stress in the early months after a baby is born. On the purely physiological level, there is quite enough change going on already. The body needs time to adjust to its new status. Rest and careful exercise combined with love and good nutrition seem the wisest course. On the psychological level, there again is a great deal of change going on. The baby has created a major life stress that demands great patience and understanding to assimilate. Additional changes create additional stress and increase the possibility of post partum depression. New parents experience a sense of the loss of freedom, the loss of their past life, as well as the loss of pregnancy and the fetus. They are challenged with accepting a new identity and discovering a new set of roles, relationships and rules within their family. All of this is going on while the infant is making its own demands on their time, energy, and emotions.

Even women who consider their overall adjustment to motherhood to be positive have moments of despair. The entire post partum period, like pregnancy, is characterized by extreme emotional responses, both good and bad. Descriptions of horrible moments often go hand-in-hand with descriptions of excitement and joy.

It is hard for new parents to keep on an even keel. It is not realistic to try to pass through the childbearing year unchanged, since there has been a major change. To achieve a more mature level, it is almost necessary to go through some upheaval. Change, even if it results in a fuller and more mature life, often produces insecurity, anger, and frustration.

Older parents may feel the intrusion of an infant

more acutely than younger parents because they are more set in their ways; but because they are older and more experienced, they have had more time to ponder the changes that may occur, and therefore are more able to cope with stress. They are sure to have experienced loss and change before. They have been through other life crises, and they have developed resources over the years for dealing with these things.

We would like to mention once again that parents have been ingenious in forming self-help groups. They range from informal meetings in someone's house to more structured early child development courses, from meetings in the park to lectures by psychologists and experts on many subjects related to parenting. Hotlines and warmlines have been set up all over the country and are used by many, so that the childbearing years for older and younger parents are made easier by many community activities.

5

THE FATHER WHO HAS WAITED SO LONG

In the course of our work, it has become obvious to us that there are few differences between the emotional responses of fathers who are well into their thirties and those who are around 25 years old. Most of what seems to hold true for older fathers applies equally well for fathers in younger age brackets. In some cases, a man's readiness to relax his work commitments and take time out to be with his wife and new child was related to his being older and in a better position to slow down, but really has more to do with the individual than with his age.

The more we learn about the feelings men have when they become fathers, the more we are convinced that men and women really confront many of the same issues at this time in their lives. The experience of becoming a *parent* overwhelms the distinctions between becoming a father and becoming a mother.

It is obvious that a man does not have a uterus and cannot be physically pregnant. Nor can he give birth or breast feed. These are momentous experiences that are unique to women and that give them a very special relationship to their bodies and their children. Nevertheless, men can get remarkably close to the transformational experience of birth. They know that the baby is genetically theirs, that its arrival will affect their lives profoundly. If they are close to their wives, they can experience the physical changes of pregnancy at very close range. Many men experience the pregnancy as being a momentous occasion in their own lives, as happening to themselves as it were. If they fail to acknowledge this truth, they may fail to accommodate to one of life's most significant events.

Pregnancy, childbirth, and parenting can be viewed as something that happens only to women. Women are capable of performing these functions alone. Children are often raised with little contact with their fathers. Most of the families with whom we talked have not wanted that to be the case for them, however. They often remarked that their own parents were distant from each other, and that all child-rearing was relegated to the mother and all wage-earning to the father. They often experienced their mothers as overprotective and their fathers as coldly distant. They have chosen to create a different way of life for themselves. Delayed parenthood, childbirth education classes, and involved fathering are often part of this decision to try to be parents in a "better" way, a way that frees the woman to follow some of her own interests outside the home and that frees the father to become involved with his children inside the home.

Men who become fathers after the age of 30 are often in a better position to become involved in their parenting than men who have their children earlier. The twenties is a period of decision-making, training, and getting started. Because most American men feel that their work forms a central part of their identity, they consider these apprenticeship years the most important of their lives. In the scramble to get the good jobs, learn the ropes, and discover a personal style in the work world, a man seldom has the emotional energy left over to invest in his other self, his family self. He may not be in a place in his career where he can afford to say "not now" to important clients or to re-arrange his schedule. He may feel an acute conflict between his personal life and his professional life.

The age of 30 does not magically change all this. Older men are often still subject to the same pressures as younger men. They may still be searching out their work identity, or just completing professional training, or not yet on a sound financial basis. Or, if they have been successful, they may well have become addicted to their work to the extent that they do not know how to relax. A man at any age can experience family demands in conflict with work demands. He must make his own personal choice about his priorities. Paternity can be carried on from a distance. This is a time-honored choice that is often made by men of all ages.

But the changes of the 1970's have created another style of fathering. We have talked with many men who are as closely invested in the process of becoming parents as are wives. Some men did not expect this to happen; others knew all their lives that it would. Thus, one man said to us, "I never really thought about it until I went to our first Lamaze class. Until then, I had just sort of assumed it was something Jane was doing. Now I'm really into it. I wouldn't have missed it for the world." In contrast, another said, "I've always wanted to have children. I was involved before she even got pregnant. As soon as I found out it was real, I flipped out and was very, very excited." This second father, the one who "always knew" that fathering would be important to him, is not alone. Men can be as committed to the seriousness of the role of father as women to the role of mother.

Many couples who have made the decision to share parenting also want to share the responsibility of earning money. They choose this path because they believe it will liberate the man as well as the woman.

> I felt we both had to have work we liked. The example of my mother was before me and influenced me. She was dissatisfied until she settled the issue of her own work outside the family, which she did not do until the three of us children were adults. I did not want the person I married to have this issue in her life. I wanted her to have work. I didn't think she was going to be happy otherwise. I wanted this for her, and for me, because I did not want to be as my father had been. I wanted to share responsibility for earning a living with someone who could help me. I didn't want all the burden on my back. I had seen that make my father dissatisfied and tense, and sick.

While the role of father is often defined by externals, by earning the money and giving the family its last name, these are not the only involvements that men can feel. When a man is intimately involved with his wife's pregnancy, the entire process can take on physical overtones for him as well as for his wife.

> When I heard she was pregnant, I became afraid I was too old to be a good father. I'm nowhere near as healthy and active as I was when I was 18. How am I ever going to be a good father? Will I be able to keep up with my kids? Will I have the strength to meet the demands of fatherhood? I made up my mind to become healthier.
> The first day, I went out to the Central Park Reservoir and jogged around. I jogged over a mile. I was relieved I was able to run that whole way. I knew then that I could be healthy enough to be a good father. I've continued to jog. I've

given up smoking, I watch my diet, and I try to be as informed about health as I can. I want to live and be healthy. I feel I have an obligation to a child and to his brothers or sisters to be a healthy parent. I also want to have life and energy left for my own life.

This man's commitment was not just for the pregnancy or for the birth experience. He was committed to an entire life as a father. He was supportive of his wife through the pregnancy, and having taken childbirth preparation classes with her, he was able to coach her in labor; he was present for the birth. But these were simply landmarks along the way. His true goal was to define himself as a father, as the kind of person he wanted to be in his own life and in his family.

Almost everything we have said about the experience of the birth and the early post partum days for women could also be said for men. Men do not undergo the same physiological changes, but if they participate in the birth, they may find that almost all of the other experiences are true for them. They are under stress and can become exhausted from lack of sleep and exhilarated from an exciting birth. They can over-identify with the baby, with their mothers, or with their wives. They also experience identity conflicts. In a more positive vein, a father can be an integral part of the birth experience. Most strikingly, he can become just as bonded and attached to his infant as his wife can.

In Chapter Three we described the encounters that take place between a new mother and her infant if they are left alone together in the early hours following the birth. Almost identical encounters occur among men who are left alone with their infants. Men, too, reach out and touch their newborn. They explore the baby's body, arms, legs, fingers, and toes. They talk and smile to it and cuddle it in their arms.

They cannot feed it milk from their breasts, but physical nourishment is only one small part of caring for a baby. The other creature comforts—the need to be loved and held, touched and soothed, talked to and smiled at—all these can be provided by the father or any other loving person who establishes a deep relationship with the baby.

Fathers who have the opportunity to be with their babies in these intimate ways are profoundly affected by the experience. They have a very different experience than fathers who choose a more traditional route.

In the past, a father was expected to take care of all the practical details. He would remain in the waiting room, or run last minute errands to buy diapers or a crib. He could phone relatives. But his involvement was indirect. The event was exciting, but its consequences were often viewed as a burden more than as a major new experience. New fathers are now discovering a closer involvement with the process.

> When Noah was born I took five weeks off. It was as if I had started on a new love affair. I lost my sense of time. I didn't really know how life passed, and when I was away from Noah I had butterflies in my stomach, and it hurt to be away from him. My life seemed as if all the building blocks had been thrown around, but they are now coming back in a new order, which seems better than the original order. I feel very responsible now. I'm more ambitious in my work. Also I drive the car much more carefully, and I even plot my strategy in the street when I am walking with the baby, especially if he is in the snuggly. I plot space physically to make him secure.

The father has traditionally been the protector. This aspect of the role has not been lost by the intimate involvement through the early weeks. These new fathers still see themselves in traditional male roles. They are wage earners; they are responsible protectors. But they also acknowledge an additional relationship to fatherhood, a relationship that is more physical and intimate. Some people still think of this as "maternal love," but we are convinced that it applies equally to both men and women.

According to our social expectations, women are supposed to love their babies right away and men are supposed to take time to get used to them. We have not found this distinction to be the case. For example, a wife remarked to us, "He's a man and they like children when they are older and can be talked with, not when they are younger and messy." When we spoke with this father himself, we found that he had no such assumption. He felt that he would and could perform any aspect of baby care, but that his wife did not seem to want him to help in certain ways. He said he almost felt *unnatural* because his love for his baby was so physical and "maternal." Some men feel comfortable with their infants instantly; some women need time to get used to them. Parental love is both fragile and complex. It can take the form of total absorption for either the mother or the father; it can also take the form of aloofness, detachment, and disengagement for either sex, but not without the loss of a potentially rejuvenating and enriching experience.

A man who achieves an intimate relationship with his child may be less conflicted about some of the things he has to give up in his life. On the most simple level, anyone in a house with a new baby can expect to give up sleep. Babies do cry in the night. It is a rare new father who can distance himself so much from the family that he can pass the nights undisturbed by the infant's needs. Many men get up in the night to bring the baby to their wives to nurse;

others change the baby's diaper or give it its bottle. They often take a paternity leave of two weeks or more and try to get as involved as possible in the changes that are occurring in their lives.

> For two weeks we were in a dream world of wonder and excitement, exhaustion and beauty, set in motion by the biological time clock of an infant's sleeping and feeding schedule. We stayed in the house, holding the baby in our arms, lying next to him when we slept, never leaving him. We couldn't forget about him for a moment. I thought he was very fragile. His life seemed precarious. I wanted to hold on to him so nothing would happen to him. I was afraid that if I left his presence, he would disappear.

Men generally return to work much sooner after a birth than women. They are still considered lucky to get two weeks leave. The return can be experienced as a time of separation and loneliness and even as one of great concern. After the period of intense togetherness, the baby has entered the father's psyche. He knows he is its caretaker. Can it survive without his presence? The man quoted above tells of his feelings:

> I reluctantly returned to work while Ann stayed with the baby for a few more weeks. Nothing happened to him while I was away. He didn't disappear. I began to see that he was a separate being from me, and with care he was going to make it. I guess I saw that I was going to make it, too.

When a man must give up his role of intimate caretaker to return to work, he may become insistent that his wife do everything "right." She becomes the extension of himself, the one who has the privilege of staying home with the baby. Ironically, many women find that they are no longer as content staying home with the baby after their husband has returned to work because they want to share in parenting equally and are frightened of being cast into the traditional role of housewife and mother.

Occasionally, career demands create a situation in which the father must take over more domestic functions than the mother. Although we have heard a great deal about this from the media, we have found that in actuality it is quite rare. Nevertheless, it does happen. A father who found himself in this situation when his son was seven months old described his experience:

> I had to learn how to take care of him. I picked up the basics in a few weeks; the rest I'm still learning. I had to learn about timing. I would come home and have some ideas that the baby had to eat, have a bath, and get put to bed at a regular hour. I always seemed to be a little off with everything. Night after night I would wind up giving a screaming, tired baby a bath. I couldn't figure it out. It infuriated me. I tensed. I thought I was doing things right and everything was coming out wrong. I finally realized I had to get ahead of his time clock. I made dinner earlier so he could eat when hunger struck. That made him happy and I relaxed. Then it was easy to be gentle with him in the bath. I had to learn how to distract him, get his attention fixed to an interest to calm him. I learned how delicate babies are. Not fragile—they don't break like a piece of crystal, but they are delicate. They are moody, and very, very passionate. When they're hungry, they're hungry; and when they're tired, they are very tired.

The things that men have to learn about infant care aren't any easier or less frustrating than the things women have to learn when they are the primary caretaker.

Couples can share parenting or one can do much more than the other. There are as many styles as there are families. The difficulty is in finding a style that is suited to the needs of all members of a particular family. During pregnancy, the needs and conflicts are still hypothetical; after the baby is born, they are real. Some months of experimentation, and even of conflict, are often required to work out a viable pattern. As all the members of the family continue to grow and change, it may be necessary to modify or even revolutionize a system that had worked well at an earlier stage. Parenting, like marriage, requires flexibility and creativity as well as love.

When a relationship has been based on companionship and camaraderie, the sudden role differences that so often appear in the post partum period can be very unsettling. Most families still find themselves relying on the mother as the primary caretaker and the father as the primary wage earner. The husband may find himself jealous of his wife's "leisure." The wife finds herself jealous of her husband's "freedom." Both can become lonely for each other in a new way.

> Ivan had taken a new job and was working longer hours than before. Then he started pressuring me to go out more; we were both feeling a lot of loss in our relationship. For him I think the breast feeding may have been one part of it. I don't think it was the major thing, but it was one more reason for him to feel locked out, like his life was changed, like his life was over. "Where is my wife, where are the old times we used to have?" And I was tired and not as interested in anything—in sex or in going out or in

our relationship or in doing little things for him. We were just drifting apart.

Many men and women have told us that they were shocked to discover how much stress the baby put on their marriages, marriages that in some cases had been firmly established for many years, even though the baby was so deeply wanted and so long awaited. They usually weren't talking about the immediate post partum period, but were thinking of the entire first year or so. The early weeks may require difficult adjustments, but they do not shake deep marital commitments. The period is recognized as a special time and everyone feels the intensity of the event. Life is new and strange. By six months later, however, the "new life" can be disturbing to both the husband and the wife.

If the baby is not an integral and positive part of the father's consciousness, he may constantly be blaming the changes in his life on his wife or on the baby itself. When he has established his own relationship with the baby and carries it with him everywhere, in his mind if not on his body, he will be more likely to be aware of the conflicts as occurring within himself rather than as occurring between himself and his wife.

> I would like to go out a little more frequently, and on the surface it seems that it should be easy to go out on a regular, if limited basis. But it isn't so simple. As we're away from home a lot working, we want to be home as much as possible also, because home has become a very attractive place. There's something happening there we don't want to miss. But we need to be free from home, too, and we try to arrange for a babysitter once a week. It's a conflict. It has taken us time to believe in our obligation to

ourselves and each other, our obligation to ourselves for relaxation and to our own relationship.

Fatigue and lack of entertainment are offset by new things. The baby gives me energy, a tremendous amount of energy. He grows before my eyes, a powerful force right in my own house, making me feel younger. This little life force teaches me much about life: he cried before he smiled, but when he smiles, it's beautiful. He's demanding, but has a way of capturing my concern. He has expanded my life, so there is more room for him.

A father who has not had the opportunity to be intimate with his infant does not get these rewards. He has all of the inconveniences, but few of the compensating joys and excitements.

Unfortunately, even an eager father does not always have a chance to establish and maintain a really close relationship with his infant. Frequently, demands outside the home make it impossible. Sometimes, the closeness of the mother-infant bond really does not allow the father in. Some mothers want to mediate every interaction between father and child.

She's so competent and good with the baby, whenever he starts to cry I hand him over to her. Of course, she can breast feed him. What can I really do to comfort him, you know?

This self-deprecating remark is typical of men who would like to become more comfortable with their infants, but feel inadequate in their ability to do what they think of as "mothering."

Some families have observed the subtle pattern through which wives train husbands to be uncomfortable with messy or fussy babies and work to maintain greater equality.

I noticed that both of the grandfathers really adore holding the baby, but as soon as he gets fussy, they hand him over to the grandmothers. It's like a double fault. Women always feel like they can take care of the baby better, so they want to take him away and then men feel like they can't do it. After noticing that, now I don't want to take the baby away from my husband when he is crying. I want Hank to feel like he can take care of him. I still feel like I can do it better, but I think that's a fallacy.

Older couples who generally have been married longer have the advantage of a deeply established trust of one another. They are likely to have learned to share in many aspects of their lives and will bring this approach to their parenting. If a father has taken the decision to be involved, there is no question in our minds that he can handle his baby with the greatest confidence.

6

MOTHERING AND WORKING

At the moment, our society values the skills of the work world over the skills of homemaking. We are generally not trained to be parents and we are not told that it is the most important occupation possible. Since the economy has made it difficult for a family to live on the income of a single wage earner, it is essential for most women to get a job outside the home. Moreover, women increasingly feel that having a job is an important and rewarding aspect of life.

Many studies of the impact of childbearing on marital adjustment have reported that highly educated and career-oriented women experience a great deal of conflict in the early years of parenting. It has also been reported that in dual-career families the husband does not experience the conflict as intensely as the wife. Even in our era of "liberation," it is women who bear the primary responsibility for children. Even when she is away from home during the week for ten hours a day, the mother is still, in all likelihood, the most important caretaker of the baby.

In spite of the clear shift to values that support the working woman, many women still feel a strong attraction to the option of staying at home with the baby. Most experience some conflict about whether or not to work, in part because there is a very strong positive pull to stay with the baby. There is also some negative pull, in the form of guilt and a sense that staying at home is what mothers are *supposed* to do.

It is inevitable that any person who fully confronts the possibility of becoming a full-time parent would experience a conflict between that role and other work. The two situations are usually mutually exclusive simply because a person cannot be in two places at once. The conflicts, however, are more than physical. Full-time infant care requires more than physical presence. It requires a special kind of deliberate approach, a particular kind of caring, patience, and gentleness. In our modern industrial society, most jobs outside the home require quite a different set of attitudes and behavior. They require paying attention to customers or clients, operating machinery, asserting opinions, making decisions, or following orders, not cooing and cuddling and feeding and nurturing. We do not live in a world that assumes women can tend their infants while contributing to the general economy.

Work often provides a sense of security for a woman who has had her job for a long time. Becoming a parent may threaten her self-esteem because of her inexperience. The situation was entirely different in the past when women considered staying at home and looking after children the most fulfilling role they could perform.

For most of the women with whom we talked, the decision to have a baby involved a conscious choice about whether to continue to work part time or full time, or whether to stop working entirely for an indefinite period. Few felt sure that they would be able to carry out their decision, however. They were uncertain what might be possible "afterwards." Many suffered a good deal of anxiety and indecision during pregnancy. In this chapter we will look at some of the choices the "older" women have made, and explore some of the conflicts that are characteristic of each choice—for we have found that no pattern is free of conflict, though some individuals pass through the period with less stress than others.

The three obvious career options for mothers are: (1) working full time outside the home; (2) working part time; and (3) having no employment outside the home. The first two of these choices necessitate that the mother rely on others to take care of her baby. She may rely on a housekeeper or babysitter who comes into the home, or an available extended family, or a babysitter outside the home (often a licensed childcare home or day-care center). The stability of childcare arrangements is a strong factor in determining whether or not a woman will be comfortable with the career option she has chosen for herself. How both the woman herself and her husband relate to the question of her working will also affect how things go. A reliable babysitter and a supportive husband can help a woman feel good about her choice to work full time or part time. If she is continually getting disapproval for her choices, she will experience more intense conflict than if everyone says that she is doing the right thing.

Staying at Home With Baby

One of the greatest opportunities presented by childbearing is that it can provide a "time out" from the "rat race" of the marketplace. That deadly label, "just a housewife," is often applied to exciting and vital human beings who are performing one of life's most challenging and important jobs while developing new and meaningful directions in their own lives. Many a woman who is forced by family circumstances to work outside the home would consider it a privilege to be able to take off a year or maybe even a decade from her job to explore other potentials and to enjoy the time out with her baby. For women in certain professions, such as computer science or other fast-moving technological areas, it is necessary to be in constant contact with new developments in their fields. They dare not take off even six months because they know they will become obsolete. For some jobs, a "time out" means retirement. For most, however, it is possible to get back into their original field or to retrain in a related, or even an entirely new, area even after quite an extended leave of absence.

Some serious career women feel that, because of their engrossment with baby and family concerns, they would not be able to function as well as they want at their jobs, and therefore they prefer not to work for a while.

> My focal point right now is this child, and my job would have to be secondary. If I taught, I would have to devote myself to the children when I could, and when I came home, just divorce myself from that. In a teaching situation you can't just do that, at least not the way I taught. There used to be calls at night and conferences on weekends. Now I have a child to take care of. I couldn't bring enthusiasm to the other job.

Obviously, a woman who can comfortably make a statement like this is one who does not feel too threatened by the role of housewife. She is not afraid of being trapped, stifled, or smothered by her role, her husband, or her child. Nevertheless, she is likely to find herself up against all the negative stereotypes before she is through her first year of full-time mothering.

Under current conditions, with the derogation of domestic roles, being a housewife involves taking a stand against social pressure. A woman who was brave enough to be a full-time mother told us:

> I really love this life. I hate people and society generally for making me feel guilty for just being a mother. I don't care that I'm staying at home and "stagnating" as everybody is saying. I don't feel I'm stagnating. I'm doing what is really healthy and good, and I've just been enjoying it thoroughly.

Taking care of a baby can enable a parent to explore new potentials. Not every parent has the time or the personal courage to exploit this opportunity for change, but some are willing to give it a try.

Many women use the time during which they are not working at a job to think about career directions. While this may not come up very much in the first three months, it can become an increasing concern as the baby grows more active and independent. The freshness of the "new life" has died down by then. The baby is probably sleeping through most nights. Solid foods are starting to provide a lot of the calories, and therefore the baby is taking less from the breast. The mother's energy level may be returning to normal. The baby is alert and conscious and seems better able to make its demands clearly known. The mother can think about other things, knowing that the baby can find her if it needs her or that it can be understood by someone who does not know it as well as she. Such a mother may decide to explore new possibilities in her own life.

> I've been a teacher for twelve years. I've been very good at it. But I also feel that I've only tapped one of the resources that is me as a

> person. I have other talents. Some of them may
> be pretty subdued, but I must be able to do
> something other than just teach. That is my forte
> in life, and I will probably continue doing it, but
> I might try something else. It may be hard to
> start something later in life, but then I'll just
> have to try harder.

As she begins to look beyond her immediate situation, a woman who has been totally absorbed in her baby may find that her environment offers very few satisfying resources. As her husband returns to full-time involvement with his job, a woman can grow increasingly lonely, especially in a suburban environment when there are no close friends or extended family nearby. This seems especially poignant for older women who have lived in the city and moved to the suburbs during the pregnancy. They have neither had time nor occasion to get to know their neighbors. They do not feel they have much in common with the women ten years younger than themselves whom they see pushing strollers to the park. Once the nesting-in period is over, a mother is more likely to be content and happy if she is in an area within reach of established friends and family. Again, it may take the ingenuity and resourcefulness of years of experience on a responsible job to have the skills to find solutions to her problems. The older woman may be more used to freedom, but she is also more used to adjusting her life to changing circumstances.

> Perhaps the women who say they're bored are
> really feeling the loss of freedom. In the first
> couple of months I felt like that, that I had this
> child and I couldn't skip around and do my own
> thing. But then I decided that I'm not going to
> be a slave to this child; she'll have to come along.

I do respect her time, but I just say, "Well, cutie, we'll just have to pack our things. Mom wants to go out."

Many older women come to remarkably creative answers when faced with the dilemma of boredom and aloneness in the middle of the baby's first year of life. Returning to work full or part time is one obvious solution, but there are many others. Some women take courses or develop creative hobbies. Others join support groups or even start their own support groups for new mothers. Some join a whole series of groups: gym or swim classes for babies, discussion groups for mothers. These classes can help the individual woman to maintain a viable sense of self and to contemplate the future.

> There is a stimulation that you miss. The support group helps because it gives you other adults to relate to instead of just being with the baby all the time. I think after being out in the work world for so many years, you are more aware of what there is out there. When you stay home you are afraid that you are losing out on something. In the group you can talk about it and rededicate yourself to this other job, the one of being a mother.

We have not talked to any full-time housewife-mothers who were not aware of alternatives. Their commitment to the role is based on a belief in the value of parenting and on a personal decision to be with the child, not on their inability to do anything else.

> I wouldn't want to miss out. The changes are so gargantuan from birth to a year. It's like the first grade, where from nothing they start to write, to read, to think. Sometimes I think about the

thousands of dollars I could be earning out there, and I look at her and I say, "Are you worth it?" That's what it's about for me. The value of it, her first year, her life. Twenty-five thousand a year can't compete with it, not for now.

When a mother is committed to the care of her baby as her primary responsibility, it does not mean that she needs to be with the child all day every day. Many "full-time mothers" have supplementary caretakers. Fathers often take over for a morning or an evening or even a day or two a week while the mother pursues things of interest to her. Grandmothers, aunts, cousins, teenaged neighbors, and professional childcare operators can all look after the baby while the mother is involved elsewhere.

Just as the babies of employed mothers can benefit from the network of caring people, the babies of full-time mothers can also benefit from a consistent experience of being with others. The tight biological bond that can be such a powerful, positive force in the early months of a baby's life must gradually give way to increasing separation and independence. Both mother and child need to discover themselves as individuals even as they maintain their awareness of the special love they have for each other. Our isolated, single-family households sometimes do not provide a healthy opportunity for babies to learn to love more than one other person. This can impoverish the life experience of both the baby and the mother.

For many older mothers who have had years of work experience, the decision not to work has been guided by courage rather than inevitability. It receives little support from society, and yet it is a very viable option that will call on all the creativity and competence of the mother. She must find sources of self-esteem and social support to provide for her own needs as well as those of her child. While not an easy career choice, the years of full-time mothering can provide an exciting time out that can shape a life in new and unexpected directions.

Working Part Time

Working part time can mean anything from spending an occasional hour or two helping out at a family business to working four full days a week in a salaried job. The impact of the job on a woman's experience as a mother will be related to the number of hours she spends on it, but also to the ease or difficulty with which she can integrate her work with her mothering.

Many of the women who work part time during the first year after they have a baby had not planned to do so when they were pregnant. The decision emerges as a result of financial need, an unexpected job opportunity, or a growing restlessness and discontent with staying at home. It often involves a combination of positive and negative motives, the attraction of job rewards and the wish to distance oneself from the housewife syndrome.

The part-time job may offer a pleasant reprieve from household chores while keeping the woman in touch with the work world. It is often even more than that. A part-time job can be a creative opportunity to explore new job possibilities. A teacher can try out what it is like to have a job in sales; a flight attendant can explore her secret ambition to be a clothing designer. A computer programmer can become a teacher's aid. When the birth of a baby has created an opportunity to give up a full-time job, it can also be a chance for change. A person who is flexible in career goals in the early years of parenting has a unique opportunity to explore new aspects of her own human potential.

Not all part-time jobs are creative. A woman working outside the home for half a day, five days a week, confronts many of the same issues as a woman working full time. She must find adequate childcare and must resolve her jealousies and guilt about leaving the baby with someone else. She must also deal with the demands and fatigue of living in two worlds at once and of working at two jobs at once. While the schedule may be extremely demanding, it can also have some inherent rewards.

Joanie is a woman who returned to her secretarial job at a government agency when her baby was three months old. She got up at seven every morning, fed the baby, put it in the playpen, showered, dressed, and ate her own breakfast, then went to work. Her husband, Jim, would still be in bed. He would stay there until the baby fussed and demanded attention. Then he would get up and take care of her. He was a writer and would try to get some work done in the morning, but would do most of his writing in the afternoon and evening. Joanie returned from work at 1:15. She gave the baby her lunch and took care of her for the rest of the day.

While Joanie's schedule was very demanding, she felt that it was also fun. She had returned to work because she and Jim needed the money, but she was looking forward to it as well:

> I like those four hours a day at the office. The people there are like a family. It's relaxing and nice and those people are all my friends. It's a good time for me. I also enjoy the walk there and back. I feel free and alone during that time.

Joanie felt that part of the pleasure in working came from its being so different from what she was doing the rest of the time. If it had not been for her job, she would have been bound to a small city apartment and a small baby all day, every day, for she would not have been able to afford an occasional or a regular babysitter. She did not feel she could have justified leaving the baby with Jim for anything less crucial than a paying job. She was considerably more content after she returned to work than she had been during the first three months of full-time mothering.

Joanie did not have any career aspirations or any desire to work full time. She thought it was much nicer to work part time than it had been to work full time. Not every part-time worker agrees. Some women take part-time positions because they feel that they should not be away from their babies full time, but really are eager to pursue their careers and feel held back by their parenting. Such a career woman is likely to bring work home with her, in her head if not in her briefcase, at the end of her official working hours. As one remarked, "I feel like I have a circuit overload. That's what it's like having a kid and trying to keep up your life."

A teacher who changed from a full-time to a part-time position in a private secondary school described the trouble she had integrating her sense of herself as a mother with her sense of herself as a professional person:

> I'm not aware of myself as a mother when I'm teaching classes. Of course I know it's there, but I'm very pleased to have this other world back. It's like my past life, like a tiny bit that I've been able to salvage. I like to forget that I'm that other person when I am in the classroom.

Perhaps part of the reason why this woman devoted her full attention to her work was because of her negative associations with the role of housekeeper-mother:

> If I was around just mothers, I would be so bored so fast, I could almost feel myself shut down and

go to sleep half way. It's like I've got to have some other part of myself functioning or I would go nuts. I didn't know that about myself before I had the baby, but when I realized it I went right back to work part time. For a while I was just hungry all the time. I realized that it wasn't for food. I was just spiritually and emotionally deprived, just so hungry.

A woman who discovers she is not happy with the role of housekeeper-mother may still feel very strongly about the importance of mothering. This means that she wants the best possible care for her child. Lori describes her philosophy:

Since I can't do that kind of interaction hour after hour, I figure the next best thing I can do is find someone who can and who likes it and enjoys it. She [the babysitter] just gets the biggest kick out of playing with him and everything, and it just bored me to tears after a while, so he responds to her positively. Then when I *am* with him, I feel more playful and not as bored.

Finding a woman who felt more content than she about caring for infants did not feel like a permanent solution to Lori. It had its inevitable drawbacks:

Her views aren't the same as mine. She has trouble saying no, and she doesn't handle anger very well. There was also a moment of guilt when he caught this cold at her house, but I suppose he would have caught it somewhere else. He's with three other little kids there during the day. If he's going to be around little kids, he's going to get sick, but then he gets the social stimulation of being around them, too.

Although she was very ambitious and career-oriented, Lori could not imagine working full time. It was simply not in her value system:

> When a woman works full time, I wonder why she did it, why she had a kid. I have certain values, certain beliefs, that I want. I have certain ways that I want him raised.

Lori's ideals of motherhood were in conflict with her "needs" to maintain her professional identity. She was aware of her dilemma even before she became pregnant. She knew that there would be conflicts, but she decided that the possible rewards would make having a baby worth the risks and the complications.

When a woman does not want to leave her baby more than fifteen hours a week but does want to receive the benefits of work outside the home, she may have to be creative in her solutions. Older women may have some advantages. They simply have had more experience in the work world. They may be more aware of job options and more able to find solutions for their domestic problems as well.

A business woman named Connie took a time-management course after her baby was born. This forced her to make conscious choices about what to do and what to eliminate. Her management experience in the business world made it relatively easy for her to "screen the market" of babysitters and child-care arrangements and to find a place where she could leave her baby three half-days a week.

Women who experience an intense need to work outside the home can also be devoted to their babies. Connie described her feelings the first day she left her baby with the sitter. "I felt so bad I could hardly breathe." Although it was painful, she felt that it was important for her to work. She had started her own graphics business just before she became pregnant. She had allowed it to dwindle to almost nothing around the time the baby was born, but she began building it back up again when he was about five months old. She managed her time by taking care of the visits to print shops and to artists while taking the baby with her and reserving the days that the baby was at the babysitter for the important meetings with clients.

Connie was very successful at running her business and caring for her baby because of the flexibility of her schedule and also because she allowed the rhythm to establish itself. She had no expectations that she could do it; she told her clients that if the work was not done before the baby arrived, she might have to turn the job over to another business. Her clients remained loyal to her and she found herself happy to pick up the work gradually. As the baby grew older, both she and the baby became more comfortable with separation. She gradually added more and more work. It was perhaps because she had been willing to drop everything that she was in fact able to keep it going. In the early months, she said, "I may not earn very much, but at least I'll keep my finger in."

Another woman had the opposite experience with her own business. She was the sole proprietor of a store. She had several employees, but no one she could trust completely to run the business for her. She was unwilling to consider the possibility of closing the business down, even temporarily, and could not find a way to delegate the responsibility to anyone else. While this situation could have worked if she had been willing to hire a full-time housekeeper, she did not consider this a viable option. It simply was not commensurate with her image of social propriety. She had never known anyone who had a housekeeper and could not imagine having another woman inside her home and caring for her baby. She tried taking the baby with her to work, but she found it to be an intolerable intrusion. Her employees were not people who could comfortably pick up a wet or squalling baby while she was busy with a customer, and she herself did not want to be patting an infant while discussing a discount. Something had to give. Predictably, it was the mother's health. When she was bedridden, she *had* to hire help. She then realized that this was a reasonable solution even under normal circumstances.

It is possible to combine childcare with managing a business, but it requires a particular kind of personality and a particular kind of business environment. To be comfortable in the two roles simultaneously, a woman has to give herself time to become fully comfortable with the baby and with herself as a mother. She can do this during the period of nesting-in. Then she may find that she can gradually move back into the business world, perhaps taking the baby with her part of the time. In a family business, this may be easier, for there may be more than one caretaker on the job. A baby can play happily in a playpen in the corner of a store if it is aware that all the people there are potential caretakers. A fringe benefit of such an arrangement is that the baby becomes attached to a larger number of people and will be content to be with them, which leaves the mother free to do other things.

Women who arrange part-time employment are often very flexible in their childcare arrangements. They are likely to rely on their husbands a great deal, either on a regular basis or to fill in for special events related to work. In general, the women who work part time do so because they want the emotional rewards that they get from the job as much or more than they want the money. They like the feeling of being away from the house and doing other things and staying in touch with the outside world. Some also feel invigorated by being away from the baby for a while. The flexibility of their jobs generally makes it possible for them to be sure that the child is being as well taken care of as if they themselves were staying alone with it all day. Babies seem to flourish under this system when the caretakers are loving, attentive people. It broadens their social network, as they become able to distinguish one person from another. Instead of developing an anxiety at being with strangers, babies who have had consistent care from a network of cooperating people seem open to new encounters and trusting of the world about them.

There are sometimes problems with childcare arrangements. It is important that the parents continue to monitor childcare arrangements and adjust them to the changing needs of the developing child. A system that worked when the baby was five months old may be inappropriate when it is twelve months old. It may seem like a nuisance to have to be continuously juggling and evaluating arrangements, but it is even more uncomfortable to have to live with an unhappy baby.

Working Full Time

Women who work full time while their children are infants generally resolve their conflicts between career and motherhood by placing their careers as a high priority and fitting the role of mother (with its increased domestic responsibilities) in to everything else they were already doing in their lives.

In some ways, the conflicts are clearest and simplest (if most intense) for women who take only a few weeks off for the birth. It may feel like an impossible decision during pregnancy, but by the time the baby is six or eight months old, most working mothers who have been able to make reasonable childcare arrangements sound confident about what they are doing. They are clear in their life choice. They may not have taken a creative leap, but they are free from the tension of ambivalence.

When a mother wants to return to work within the first six weeks after the baby is born, she will probably need to have a babysitter who comes into the home and does some housework as well as childcare. Many women, particularly if they are nursing, continue to experience quite a bit of fatigue for the first two months. Most babies are still waking up during the night and may be quite fretful at this stage. A full-time job plus household and infant responsibilities is too much for most women unless they have a small, easy-to-care-for apartment, a relaxed baby, and a very helpful husband. A full-time housekeeper is indispensable for a woman who wants minimal disruption of her lifestyle and who wants her career to go on as before. But such a solution is generally based on economic need and may not apply to many women even if they are older and have established careers.

A woman may underestimate the fatigue she will experience if she pushes herself too far. Several women have told us that they wish they had worked until later in the pregnancy and had taken an extra week or two off afterwards, simply so they could be more thoroughly rested.

The initial adjustment may still be difficult. At one month post partum, most women still feel tired and vulnerable. They may feel defensive, especially in a male-dominated field. One woman said: "I tell my colleagues just to pretend I had a heart attack if they are annoyed that I missed a committee meeting or was late with a report."

Career women are not necessarily unloving or unfeminine or unmaternal. They have the option of remaining childless, and choose to have babies because they want them. Thus, one of the conflicts inherent in their choice is whether or not to leave the baby with someone else all day.

> There's a tug, a tug for the baby, between me and the housekeeper, and its kind of funny, I mean he is my baby. I'm very glad I'm nursing. I wouldn't have had it any other way. I recommend it for anyone who is leaving their baby during the day, because I know he knows me and that I'm indispensable. When I come in at lunch time, he's waiting and that's really nice. The housekeeper is more secure with him and handles him better. I'm glad I have someone I can trust. But there is that tug.

We also met a career-oriented woman who found the "tug" so great that she gave up her job and stayed home for the first three years. There can be a strong positive pull to be with the baby. Many dedicated career women, however, feel that the role of housewife-mother is not for them. Career women are often very assertive, high-energy women with strong needs to achieve things in the outside world. They may have an image of another self they might wish to be—a gentle, patient, all-giving, self-sacrificing mother —but they know that this is not who they are. Several have made remarks almost exactly like the following:

> Sometimes I wonder why I don't just stay home and take care of the baby. But I know the answer. It's because I'd probably go out of my mind, that's why.
> I could give up work, you know, *working*, in a minute. But it's the psychic pleasure, the rewards of being recognized for being good at something—that's what would be difficult to give up. Nobody's going to write me a memo saying,

"That was an outstanding job you did overcoming his resistance to sleep last night...."

The woman who takes a very short leave from work essentially integrates her maternal identity with her professional identity from the very beginning. She faces fatigue and may experience a very intense period of stress, but essentially her conflicts are soon over—assuming she can make a reasonable child-care arrangement.

It is far more common for working women to take an extended maternity leave of three months, six months, or a full year, than for them to return to work in the first month. The great advantage of the extended leave is that it does give time to recuperate physically and to adapt to the role of being a mother. There is more time to develop a sense of the self as protector and provider for the baby.

> I was all for going back after three months, but the more reading I've done the more I've thought about it. The baby is just so small that I don't want to leave her yet. At six months, she'll be starting to sit up, she'll be more independent. It'll be easier to leave then.

There is probably no truly "easy" time to leave a much-loved baby, but there are times of greater or lesser vulnerability—not only for the baby, but also for the mother—just as there is a sense of readiness that makes a woman decide to have a baby in the first place. There can also be a "readiness" that lets a mother know when it is time to return to work. Without this sense, the return will probably be unhappy and filled with conflict. Many women who thought they would not work while their children were young found themselves on the job within the first year because they "felt ready."

An extended maternal leave allows a woman time

to assimilate her identity as someone's mother. When this happens, some women feel that the other self, the one who held a job, is very far away or even gone forever.

> It was really strange, going back to work at six months. I was afraid. I was nervous about how I would feel. I was looking forward to it, but I didn't know how I'd feel, whether I'd be guilty about leaving my baby. All the women I had been seeing over the past few months were women who were staying home with their children, and they were all telling me how nice it was to stay home, and I was getting all these negative images about going back to work.
> I had to adjust. It was as though I was coming back from my first day at work, almost like I was starting a new job. I was very nervous. I was a different person. I was Jeannie's mommy coming back to work, but I was also becoming myself again, Fran Ellis and not Jeannie's mother.

A woman who tries to do her job "just like before" but who does not get enough help at home may find herself in a very difficult situation. It is possible to work and be the mother of an infant, but it is not easy. It can only be accomplished by evaluating realistically what needs to be done and by taking responsibility for getting someone to do it. Trying to do both jobs without the benefit of help can lead to doing neither job well enough.

Sometimes a woman's sense of pride or social obligation can lead her to see the baby as only one of a long line of "demands" being made on her time and energy. There are so many *unavoidable* demands during this first year with a baby that it is hard to understand why a woman must perform *avoidable* jobs, especially if she is earning a full salary and can hire someone else to take care of the more time-consuming and routine chores. Cooking and shopping cannot always be postponed or relegated to someone else, but there are certain traditionally female jobs that can—most particularly, the kind of work involved in entertaining company or in writing "thank you" notes. Working mothers have been known to stay up until two or three o'clock in the morning to send off Christmas cards, to get up again at four to nurse the baby, and again at seven to make breakfast and go off to work. Surely, such a situation is unnecessary and irrational. It may be very important to establish priorities, and some traditional tasks may have to fall to the wayside, at least for awhile.

It is especially difficult for many middle-class American women to accept the idea of leaving their babies with someone else. The use of their own mother as babysitter is often acceptable when any other caretaker would not be. It also helps if the husband (or some other close relative) is a person who can fill in totally in case of emergency or difficulty. Many working mothers feel that their jobs fit their style of mothering and make life better for them. A flight attendant told us:

> I really like my work. I always did want to fly, and I like talking to people. When I'm flying, I can go into my room, close the door, and go to sleep just like that. When I'm home I'm always thinking of so many things that have to be done. Flying is a good break for me. I need that. I like the exposure to new things, and don't want to be shut out from the world. Other people may just fall right into the old motherhood routine, but I don't.

When she was not working, this woman felt she had nothing in common with the women around her. She did not like the image of herself as a suburban housewife. When she returned to her work as a flight attendant, she found other women who were adjusting to motherhood in a similar way, which was very reassuring for her. She felt sure that her job would turn out to be good for her daughter. She loved her own mother, but felt that she had provided a very poor role-model because she had remained a submissive housewife who never reached out to enjoy life for herself.

We hear a lot about the demise of the extended family. Nevertheless, it still does exist for many people. Parents often use their families for childcare. For a woman, this may mean her husband or an aunt or grandmother. When it is the husband or another close family member who lives in the same household, there is the advantage of the baby being able to stay in its secure environment. In addition, the mother does not have to pack up diapers and bottles and paraphernalia that seem to accumulate around babies. The adult who is caring for the child will also have time to take care of some other domestic chores. Often, however, the extended family lives somewhere else. Many mothers drop their babies off at the home of their mother or mother-in-law for the day. This arrangement generally does not create the same emotional tension that we sometimes find when mothers leave their babies with people whom they do not fully trust. There is quite a bit more flexibility in arrangements, and there is the likelihood that childcare values will be very much the same. Such an arrangement can work very well indeed during the first year.

A woman named Dorothy was leaving her baby with her mother-in-law before work and picking him up on her way home. She talked about the changes in her life created by having a baby:

> The main difference for me now that I have him is that I can't wait to get home to him. I just say,

"Oh, it's five o'clock, I have to pick up my little baby," and I go right home. He's changed my life, but I think for the better.

Occasionally we hear about a situation in which both the husband and the wife have full-time jobs and divide the time they devote to caring for the child by working separate shifts. While this situation may work out for some schedules, it means that the parents have little time to see each other or to relax and enjoy their home life. Time pressure is one of the greatest complaints of working mothers. It is not much alleviated by the husband and wife splitting up the day. The more adults (or responsible older children) there are around to share the domestic and childcare responsibilities, the less pressure on the parents. When there are several caretakers in close relationship to the baby, the mother and father have the security of knowing they will be able to get out together from time to time. They will still be responsible for their own children, but they will not forfeit all of their personal freedom to the demands of the infant.

Many women feel that when they return to work, their relationship with their husband returns to almost what it was before the baby was born. This seems more likely to occur when there is the money to afford domestic help so that the wife's working does not overburden the husband or put extreme household responsibilities on both partners. When a marriage is based on a sense of sharing, the pattern of sex-role differences that is usually assumed in the first year—in which the mother tends the baby and the father supports the family—can be unsettling. For example, one woman who remained at home while her husband was working full time was annoyed to find herself taking care of little household problems, such as broken dishwashers, cluttered garages, and dead light bulbs. She recognized that it was only fair, but she did not like it very much. After she herself returned to full-time work, she and her husband shared the responsibilities jointly. She was much more comfortable dividing the housework than doing it herself. She also liked being able to talk with her husband about his work and to share her own business ventures with him. This had always been an important part of their marriage; they did not want to lose it.

It is possible to have a baby and continue in a career with minimal disruption. In such a situation, the mother's role becomes closer to what was traditionally regarded as the father's role. She must delegate the responsibility of childcare to someone else for long periods of the day, but she will be adding to her self-image the concept of herself as a mother. She will have plenty of opportunities for mothering in the mornings, evenings, and through the long nights. It may be hardest for her to find time to relax and do things for herself. It helps if her work environment is accepting of her family roles and if her family is accepting of her outside work.

Some women feel uneasy about letting the two worlds of mothering and work overlap. While it is sometimes true that the work environment may be hostile to the idea of motherhood, it seems quite often that it is the woman herself who is unable to integrate the two parts of her life. Often the people at work can help her feel more comfortable about her situation.

> One day I took the baby to a staff meeting. I wanted to go to the meeting at nine, but I had to have him at the doctor's by ten, so I just took him with me to work. Everybody was just saying "Oooh," and they gave him a standing ovation. They just played with him and he was great. My boss was uncomfortable about it, but everybody else thought it was fine.

When the two worlds do not have to be excluded from each other, the mother can integrate her roles more easily and feel more secure in both situations.

The only real difficulties that a career woman with a baby may face are emotional. Possible feelings of jealousy may make it hard for her to retain a single, loving caretaker, and feelings of guilt may lead her to try to do everything herself instead of delegating responsibility wisely. In some cases she may lose out on some of the exciting possibilities for personal growth and joy that come from deep contact with a developing child.

The child needs consistent care by warm, attentive persons. To provide this care, the mother does not need to be the only person to care for the baby. She herself will be able to be warm and attentive only if she is happy with her life and her domestic and professional roles. Even mothers with unbroken career commitments generally find themselves the primary caretaker except when they have specifically decided to delegate that authority to someone else.

The childbearing year is a time of personal change and growth. A woman can either experience this as an interruption of her career and other interests, or she can use it as an opportunity to move in new directions. In all likelihood, she will experience it both as a distraction from her goals and as an enrichment and intensification of her life. There is likely to be some degree of conflict between the desire to continue to be active in the outside world and the desire to be a good mother. Although the conflict may sometimes become intense and uncomfortable, it may also lead to personal growth through which the mother achieves an integrated awareness of herself as both a competent and a nurturing person.

7

TIME FOR MORE?

A great deal of thought goes into an older couple's decision about whether or not to have a child. We have found that even more thought may go into the question of whether or not to have more children.

Some couples have told us about their decision to have just one child. They have experienced some pressures from friends and from their families to give their baby a little brother or sister, but they have chosen to go against convention. This was not a matter of age or a fear of physical complications. Rather, we found they based their choice on their own feelings about the importance of being good parents to the child that they had.

> I felt I could not really share my love. I knew I could do a good job with one, but I did not think I would be able to be as good a parent as I wanted to be if I had more than one. I did not realize this until after the baby was born. In fact, I had always assumed I would have more and surprised myself in feeling so strongly about it.

We have also talked with couples who decided to have a larger family.

> We enjoyed Jonathan so much that we couldn't wait to have another. I thought I might have

trouble conceiving this time, so we did not use contraceptives at all after he was six months old. I had such a good time with the first and am looking forward to the birth of the second. So far the pregnancy hasn't been tiring me out too much. My husband is absolutely delighted because he has gotten so much pleasure from the first, but he says that *no* baby will ever be as good as Jonathan.

An older woman often feels that she cannot just sit around and wait until she feels "ready" again. If she wants to have more than one, she may feel that she has to act immediately rather than allow a generous space between her children. Obviously, this is a less pressing issue for a woman in her early thirties. As a factor, it becomes most pronounced after the age of 37, even if the first experience has been a happy one.

The couples we have talked with have generally realized that their jobs would be affected by the birth of their children. Some have said that they limited the number of children in their family to reduce the years in which they would be fully involved with pre-school children.

A larger family means increased physical as well as emotional demands. Every new child is a unique addition. At the same time, the older child may be going through emotional upheavals of its own as it tries to adjust to the new baby in the house. This adds to the adjustments that the parents must make.

In our experience, older couples seem to make a greater effort to learn from their mistakes than younger couples. If they feel that they have not worked things out perfectly the first time around, they change the way they do things for the second child. Thus, a woman who did not take off enough time after her first birth will make sure to get more rest after her second. A woman who had planned to stay home full time with her first child, but found that she did not like this situation, will be more likely to make early arrangements for continuing at least part-time work after the birth of her second.

Even very thoughtful, mature, and well-organized parents cannot predict all the changes that will occur with the birth of a new child. They will have to go through a period of trial and error to find what works best for them in their new family constellation. This is as true for the second child as it was for the first.

Epilogue

One of the comments we hear most often from couples, but especially from women who have delayed childbearing until their thirties or forties, is that they lack models to show them what it will be like to be parents after such a long period of childfree adulthood. In this book, we have focused on the experience of the pregnancy and the early months of parenting, rather than present an overview of the entire life experience. We could not have done otherwise because the trend towards starting a family after 30 did not exist until very recently. However, there have always been individuals who have followed this path. We thought our readers might enjoy the stories of the authors of this book.

MY STORY
by Elisabeth Bing

It seems that one of the most difficult things for me to do is to sit in front of my typewriter and talk about myself, but I very much want to write this chapter. Not only was I "biologically" (as someone euphemistically put it the other day) an old mother, but naturally I kept on being an "old mother" right through our child's infancy, into his grade school years, through high school, and finally into his adulthood. Now, at this point in our lives, the generation gap has narrowed, and we, parent and child, find that as adults we enjoy each other's company. We have great respect for each other, laugh together, and often read the same books, but in addition we have this extraordinary bond, the bond between parent and child.

All our lives we are someone's child, belonging to a mother and a father through a bond that never seems to be broken. I know that it has never faded within me, though I am well into middle age.

The question I have often asked myself is this: When do we really grow up and become independent from those who nurtured us? I meet my brothers and sisters these days, and our relationship, our way of talking to each other, is almost the same as it was so many years ago when we were all children. I am still number 4, the child who, in the minds of my siblings, still has to be helped with so many things—with homework, with music lessons—the child who still rides to school on the handlebars of her older brother's bicycle because she isn't allowed to have her own yet.

I cannot remember ever wondering how old my parents were. I only saw them in relation to me or my brothers and sisters. They were THEY, and I was their daughter. I am still their daughter.

I was 40 years old when I gave birth to Peter. We wanted him a great deal. No, we had wanted a child to make our family complete. We did not know we would give birth to Peter; we would have accepted a Claudia just as readily. It was not really by design that Fred and I started the family so late in our reproductive lives. We had married late in life, when we were both 36 years old.

Fred had a good job, and I was establishing myself as a childbirth educator in New York. I had emigrated to the United States not long before we met, having spent the war years in England and the postwar years partly on the Continent and partly in England, trying to make my way. So my marriage to Fred meant a real settling down, almost like coming home. I had a real bedroom to sleep in for the first time in my adult life. No more sleeping on the living room couch. This felt like wonderful security. I loved it, and I wanted more; I wanted us to have a child.

And I was getting older and was well aware of the diminished chances of even getting pregnant, and of the increased possibilities of giving birth to a child with Down's Syndrome; though at that time, we did not know nearly as much as we do now; there was no chance for us to make sure of a healthy child by having an amniocentesis done. (This reassuring procedure was not available twenty-four years ago.)

Actually, it rarely occurred to me that I might give birth to a handicapped child. My most immediate worry was to get pregnant, and after trying for over one year, we sought help. We went through all the recognized treatments: Fred's sperm was more than adequate; I had my tubes blown through and X-rayed; I was put on a diet of enormous amounts of orange juice; we kept temperature charts for coitus. Our lovemaking often became somewhat less than spontaneous.

I became pregnant four times, only to miscarry very early in pregnancy. We had started making enquiries about adoptions, only to find that here too we would have difficulties, not because there were no children available, but because we were too old to be given a baby. They would only give us an older child.

And then, finally, my doctor suggested a D & C (dilatation and curettage), a common procedure after a miscarriage to make sure that the uterus is clean and that there are no fetal tissues left. I became pregnant again, carefully tiptoeing through the first three months, when every little sensation in my abdomen and belly made me extremely anxious. But I was still pregnant after three months, which had never happened before. We were blissfully happy.

The rest of my pregnancy was decidedly uneventful (a term used by the medical profession when there is nothing too interesting to take notice of). But that was exactly what we wanted, and it pleased us enormously. The more "uneventful" the better.

I found pregnancy exhilarating. I grew bigger and bigger and felt better and better. I had not felt so well, content, peaceful, tranquil, devoid of anxiety for years. Our relationship changed subtly, since we did not have to worry about becoming pregnant any more. Here we were walking around with big bellies. I say "we," because I felt Fred would almost have liked to have had a bigger belly too, simply to show how proud and happy and relieved he was.

I don't think there was a moment throughout my whole pregnancy when I was not delightfully conscious of my pregnant body. I watched it carefully, and feeling the first butterfly-like movements of the baby was a milestone during the nine months of waiting.

At the time, I was teaching childbirth classes at Mount Sinai Hospital, and I felt and knew that my teaching was changing. It had become almost personal, as if I were teaching myself and was sitting on the floor with the other women listening and taking it all in, making mental notes of what I thought would be useful in my labor, fantasizing about labor, and frequently dreaming of our child. I was just one of "my pregnant mothers" even though I was their instructor. There was no real ambiguity in that, only a happy feeling of learning and teaching at the same time.

Fred had a wonderful way of persuading me not to get too anxious about the "due date." He kept on repeating to me over and over again, "You're going to be two weeks late, you're going to be two weeks late!" so that by the end of the ninth month I was quite convinced that I was going to be two weeks late.

When I went for what I thought would probably be the second-to-last check-up, the doctor said, "I think the baby will be here within twenty-four hours; you are effaced, and have started to dilate." I simply didn't believe him, just went home and said to myself, "Oh, he doesn't know that it's going to be two weeks late. I forgot to tell him!"

Of course, he was absolutely right. The following night I woke up with slight cramps and some staining, and by the next morning when we called the doctor he said, "Come over, I'm already at the hospital."

Things happened so fast, I could hardly keep up with them. I had been in active labor for not much more than one hour when the doctor examined me and found me fully dilated and told me to push the baby out. At that point I needed help; I did not seem to get the baby down. The doctor used forceps, and I pushed, and within a very short time there was Peter.

I learned an important lesson at that point: this labor was nothing like the fantasy labor I had had for weeks. This had been reality, and I saw how important it is for a woman to work with each contraction as it occurs and to deal with the present situation, instead of becoming confused because labor does not seem to follow a preconceived pattern.

Fred stayed with me for a long time, and we had our Peter with us all the time because our hospital had "rooming in," which was a wonderful arrangement and very rare at that time in any New York hospital.

One night, though, I had a disconcerting experience. The night nurse came in, woke me up to nurse the baby, took one look at me, and said "Don't you ever wear make-up?" Then next morning she came by once more and said, "You don't seem to be nearly as old as I thought you were."

I had not thought of myself as being old or looking so old, but obviously for the night nurse I was an "old" mother, and it took me a little while to tell myself that my own feeling about myself was right for me: I felt like Peter's mother.

Soon after, I left the hospital and went home with our little Peter. What wonderful days, what unexpected, tiring days! Anxieties, fears, loneliness, and overwhelming love for the baby followed each other, or occurred all at the same time.

Having heard the reports of my students about the post partum period, the "fourth trimester," I was aware that it was no different for me. Fred was a great help, getting up in the middle of the night, changing the little one, and bringing him to me in bed to nurse. Fred would snore within seconds of having delivered him to me, and I spent a peaceful thirty to forty minutes cuddled up with Peter, nursing him, holding him, and loving him.

Both Fred and I cherished every moment of our life with Peter. We seemed to develop a way of talking to each other that took his presence into account.

When we spoke of things, we prefaced them with "that was before Peter" or "that was after Peter was born." We soon decided to just say "B.P." and "A.P." It was a very special period in our lives.

Within about three weeks I was back at the hospital, teaching. Part time, of course, just a few hours a week, and I suddenly realized that I resented being away from the baby, that it was actually physical pain I felt when I was not with him. When this overwhelming feeling occurred, I considered, for the first time, how I could make the most of my time with Peter and not waste any of it, because I would be 60 years old when he was 20. I wondered what I would be like physically and mentally when I reached that age.

Fred must have thought about that, too. One Sunday he took Peter out by himself in the park. A strange man looked at Fred, looked into the carriage, looked at Fred again, and finally said, "Father or Grandfather?" Fred came home and was quite indignant. Surely, he did not look that old! He could very easily play baseball with his son now. It couldn't be that different in a few years' time! He had never doubted it for a moment. In fact, it had never occurred to him even to think about it. But the doubts had come with the stranger's question, and they forced him to look at himself and find out how old an "old father" can be.

Soon we had established a working, caring, playing routine with Peter. This child was now part of our life, and if we could not go to so many concerts or movies or theatres, we certainly did not miss them very much.

I was dreading the idea of taking Peter to the park and having to sit day after day with him. Here I was 40 years old, and I would have to sit with all the other twenty-five year old mothers and try and make friends.

At the time I was still thinking that one could only make friends with women of one's own age. Actually, of course, we had long-established friendships with people who were our peers, our generation, and I should not have felt uneasy about having to make new friends. However, I was very worried that the other young mothers in the park would not accept me, and perhaps not accept my child.

What actually happened was that I got on famously with the younger women. The great common bond, our babies, was easily enough to bridge the gap of our ages. Very soon I stopped being self-conscious about being "an old lady of 40," because nobody else seemed to be bothered by it. The amazing thing, and very unexpected for me, was that the talk between the mothers was not only about babies. In fact, here was a group of intelligent young women who were interested in many things I was interested in. Admittedly, I did not make lasting personal friendships during this period, but this lack of intimacy never really bothered me too much. Peter was entirely accepted, whatever the age of his parents; his "years in the park" were exciting and full of friends. And that was what mattered.

In retrospect, I wonder why I even thought I would have to make strong personal attachments to other mothers. Surely, we had many friends, and I was rarely lonely. But in retrospect I can also understand that I wanted to be like the others and was afraid of being rejected because I was older, not one of them, had not been to the same schools, and already firmly established in my career. But if I was further in my career than they were, as mothers we were equals. That is to say, I was as inexperienced, as full of anxieties, joys, and love as they were.

When Peter was a year old, Fred's mother came to live in the same apartment house and that was how we got our "built-in" baby-sitter. A great love affair developed between the child and his grandmother. I always feel that grandparents are the most wonderful invention for children. And it works both ways. With three generations living under one roof, there is a sense of continuity which brings with it joy and freedom. There were also many difficult times, of course, when Fred and I had to cope with two generation gaps at the same time.

Peter's school years were busy ones. Fred and I both worked, though my work was easily arranged to leave me free for Peter the moment he came home from school and for the rest of the day. We also arranged who would supervise Peter's homework or help with certain school subjects. For mathematics, Peter had Fred and Oma, his grandmother, to help him. He could come to me for languages and literature. And finally, I also helped him with his piano practice.

We both wanted Peter to grow up with a love of music, but when he was little and I tried to encourage him to play the piano, I failed miserably. Now, that might happen to any mother at any age, but here was something I really felt I didn't have the stamina for: I could not keep up an argument with him when he did not want to practice; he wore me out, and I gave in. I always felt that was because I got more easily tired at 48 than I might have had I been 28 years old.

There was another thing I could not do with him. Peter certainly tried hard to make me go with him to baseball games. When I declined, politely but firmly, he said, "Oh, Mum, you can come, don't think you are too old. There are old women at the stadium in wheelchairs, and they enjoy it!"

When Peter was 8 or 10 years old, he said to me from time to time, "Mum, why don't you dye your hair, you'd look younger." I started going grey when I was in my thirties, and by the time Peter became aware of what I looked like, I had certainly a great deal of white hair. But then, luckily he saw one of my best friends, who had suddenly changed the color of her hair from brown to blond. Peter looked at me and said, "Don't you ever do that to your hair, Mum!"

My professional life became more demanding from year to year. I had made a rule that I would always be there when Peter got home from school, and our weekends were family weekends. Our schedules seemed to work out wonderfully. As Peter lived his own life more and more independently, I had more chances to travel and work away from home.

We three also traveled together whenever we could, and I don't think we ever had the feeling of not being able to keep up with our son.

Years went by, and Peter went to college. We took him there, and leaving him, really for the first time in our lives, was one of the great traumas for both Fred and me. Driving back home, after we said goodbye to him, we felt devastated. There should be counselors for parents when they take their child or children to college to live away from home for the first time. And that goes for older parents especially. What made us so unhappy was not that we had taken him to college, but that it was another huge milestone in our lives. It overwhelmed me to think that actually from now on Peter was really only going to be a guest in our house whenever he came home.

I'm sure most parents feel a great sense of loss when they take their child to college for the first time. I think it was especially hard on us, partly because we had only this one child and were returning to an empty and very quiet house, but mainly because we were both 58 years old and had suddenly become very aware of our age. We both felt that new periods in life, which may have been welcome and exciting steps when we were younger, had now become much harder to adjust to.

In American society growing old has always been a dreaded part of life. I think that both Fred and I were helped enormously through middle age by having a young child around, who forced us to live and share his young life with him. Actually, we never felt we were forced by him. It seemed an absolutely organic development for both of us as parents, and I am almost sure it was for Peter as well. Perhaps it is one of the great advantages of having a child later in life that the transitions one has to make are gentler and therefore easier to accept.

There was no generation gap when Peter and I spent two weeks traveling through Burgundy last summer, visiting one Romanesque church after the other, eating delicious goat cheese and drinking Burgundy wine. We were two people who enjoyed each other's company and talked on the same wavelength.

In a few months, Fred is going to meet Peter in Europe, and the two men will travel together for a while. I know that their bond and friendship is not limited by the difference in their ages.

Growing with our son, whom we had so late in our lives, has made our own lives immeasurably rich.

AND WHAT IT MEANT FOR ME
by Peter Bing

My mother and father were 40 when I was born, and I am their only child. Did their unusual age influence my development? Would I have been different if my parents had been younger? And if so, how? These are hard questions to answer—probably much harder for a son than for either parent. After all, a child's character is formed largely in the first seven years, and at that time I lacked the self-awareness to reflect on things around me. So, if there was a difference early on, I was unaware of it.

I must have been 9 or 10 when I first became conscious of my parents' age. I was playing tennis with my mother, scattering the balls every which way (at that point I could hardly keep a ball in play), and Mom went chasing about, trying to retrieve them. Ever since I can remember, Mom has had white hair. From a distance she looks a lot older than she is. So, on that day, a considerate young man came over to the fence by the court and shouted, "Hey, sonny, don't make your grandma run so much!" I was surprised. "That's not my grandma!" I replied. "That's my Ma!"

On the whole, though, I didn't think about my parents' age. None of my friends' parents were so young that I was confronted with the difference. And both Mom and Dad were physically so active they usually seemed younger than the parents of my friends. I always played catch with Dad, and he never admitted that his hands ached from my fastballs. Mine certainly did from his. I always winced as they came towards me. If anything, my parents' own consciousness of their age sometimes made *me* conscious of it. My mother's refrain after her daily yoga was, "Not bad for an old lady, eh?" But "old" was like a joke, and I had to agree: I couldn't do most of those exercises.

No, in growing up, my parents' age seemed natural to me. I never considered the advantages of younger parents or the disadvantages of older parents. On the contrary, my mother and father insisted on the rightness of their age. I soon thought that anyone who married before 30 must be crazy. What could they know of the world? How far could they have developed? What kind of security could they have? Meet as many interesting people as you can; learn and grow from them before tying yourself down. These are my parents' thoughts, but they've penetrated my blood. If a girlfriend of mine so much as mentions marriage, I become tense, and some relationships have even broken up because of this. Marriage at the age of 24, 25, or even 28 seems inconceivable. And when friends my age get engaged, I do my best to talk them out of it. This attitude simply reflects how my parents asserted their lifestyle in bringing me up. But I sometimes wonder if such a deep-seated feeling about marriage won't continue *after* I'm 30. This occasionally worries me.

On looking back, I realize how strongly and successfully my parents influenced me, and I'm certain that much of their success in this was due to their age. Both had lived through a depression and a world war, left the land they'd grown up in, lived in several countries, and worked at various jobs. On deciding to have a child, they brought experience and maturity with them. I'm sure a good deal more thought went into my upbringing than would have been the case if my parents had been 25 years old. And, as I was an only child, their concern was that much greater.

Because we lived in New York, they could expose me to most of the things they had grown up with in Germany—classical music, theatre, art, and so forth—and they did so systematically, in a way that would have been difficult outside such an unusual city. They could even send me to the Rudolf Steiner School, a school based on the European tradition. Moreover, we traveled to Europe every few years, so there was never the cultural gap that might easily arise between people separated by forty years and two cultures.

I often turned to my parents for company and friendship as a child because I didn't have brothers or sisters. Of course, I had friends my own age, but there were never the crowds of children that gather in a home where there are a number of siblings. I've heard this from other "only" children as well: they are often as close to people of their parents' generation as to those of their own. My parents' friends were mostly their age, and like my parents, were for the most part mature, experienced, financially secure, and serious about what they were doing. The wild days of their youth were past, and they had ripened into very interesting, amusing people. I enjoyed them. I looked up to them, respected their thoughts, and wanted to be like them.

Among my friends, I'm regarded as stable and reliable: a "rock of Gibraltar." I study hard and like it. If friends need help or advice, they come to me. On looking back, I'm certain that these qualities came largely from close ties to my parents and their friends. Their experience allowed me to skip much of the garbage young people wade through, and I'm grateful for this. The only problem is a lack of occasional madness. Sometimes I'm so damned sensible, I can't stand it!

Ever since elementary school, my emotional outlet has been the stage. And there, all those emotions are perfectly in place. In a strange way my upbringing made a good actor out of me. And that's an excellent way to compensate for the disadvantages of sanity. In short, my parents' age may have caused some inhibitions, but the positive effects were far more significant.

A purely practical awareness of my parents' age has come to me only in the last few years. I was in my senior year of college, when I realized that my mother and father were over 60, on the threshold of old age. I was planning to go on to graduate school, and had no thoughts of settling down or getting a job. They were still supporting me. I wondered how much longer they'd be able to work. I was afraid that perhaps I was being selfish, taking away large sums of money for my education when I was not even sure they had provided for themselves. Both my mother and father are self-employed. When they retire they'll have no pension to speak of. On the other hand, they can keep on working as long as they want or are able.

Last summer, my father had a heart attack. That brought home to me how mortal my parents are. Even if all through my childhood and adolescence into young adulthood I did not worry about my parents' age, it concerns me greatly now—all the more so because we are such close friends.

A FEW REMARKS
by Libby Colman

Both Elisabeth and Peter make it very clear that parents can be creating a healthy and wonderful life for themselves and for their children when they start their family later in life. I found the same thing to be true.

Like Peter, I grew up with parents who were more than a decade older than the parents of my friends. Also like Peter, I think that this added to their maturity and to their wisdom, and therefore made life better for me. I always thought my parents were "special." They were more even-tempered and sensible than other parents, largely because they were older.

Unlike Peter, I was not an only child. My parents married when they were 30. They had their first child when they were 34, their second when they were 36, and their third (me) when they were almost 38. I think they had only intended to have two children and had been worried about having a retarded child the third time around, but it doesn't seem to have happened.

As I was growing up, we were very much the all-American family. Our parents were as energetic and involved as any we knew—more involved than most. They treasured family life more than any others I remember. We kids all knew that Mom had supported herself for years. I always like the idea that she knew how to be successful in the work world and that she had devoted herself to family life while we were young.

The only disadvantage of having older parents that I can think of struck me when Arthur's and my children were small. They were born in my late twenties and early thirties. Soon after the second was born, my father's health began to fail. By the time our youngest son was 3½, both my parents were dead. They both died before they were 70, which is quite young, but I must admit that I'm jealous when I see children who have vigorous grandparents just turning 60. The offspring of older parents may have to be taking care of two dependent generations at once, one that is busy being born, the other that is busy dying. This is a risk, but one well worth taking. I needed top-quality parenting much more when I was 5 than when I was 35.

On the whole, people are living long enough these days to be assured that they will be able to see their own children into adulthood even when they delay parenting well past 30, though it is true that they may miss out on the pleasures of having three generations alive at the same time, especially if the second generation delays as well.

It always seemed to me that my parents believed, with Elisabeth, that their children "made their lives immeasurably rich." They enjoyed having us, and we enjoyed having them. They also continued to enjoy each other. This pleasure is the greatest legacy they have left me. I believe that it was created, in part, by their being a little older than most couples when they started their family.

Bibliography

PREGNANCY AND BIRTH

Caplan, Frank. *The First 12 Months of Life.* New York: Bantam Books, 1978.
(A well-organized account of the first twelve months, with photographs.)

Chabon, Irwin. *Awake and Aware.* New York: Delacorte Press, 1966.
(The psychoprophylactic method of childbirth and its history.)

Cherry, Sheldon H. *Understanding Pregnancy and Childbirth.* New York: Bantam Books, 1973.
(A description of pregnancy, labor, and delivery.)

Colman, Arthur and Libby. *Pregnancy: The Psychological Experience.* New York: Bantam Books, 1977.
(Feelings and experiences of expectant parents.)

Elkins, Valmai H. *The Rights of The Pregnant Parent.* New York: Waxwing Productions, 1976.
(How to communicate with doctors and hospitals to have a satisfying birth experience.)

Kramer, Rita. *Giving Birth.* Chicago: Contemporary Books, 1978.
(Childbearing in America today.)

McCauley, Carole S. *Pregnancy After 35.* New York: Dutton, 1976.
(Medical and other issues that may interest the older parent.)

Nilsson, Lennart et al. *A Child Is Born.* New York: Delta, 1966.
(The development of the fetus in beautiful photographs.)

Price, Jane. *You're Not Too Old To Have A Baby.* New York: Farrar, Straus and Giroux, 1977.
(A personal account of the experience of an older parent combined with interviews with other parents.)

CHILDBIRTH PREPARATION

Bing, Elisabeth. *Six Practical Lessons For An Easier Childbirth.* New York: Bantam Books, 1977.
(An illustrated guide to the Lamaze Method of childbirth.)

———. *Moving Through Pregnancy.* New York: Bantam Books, 1976.
(Exercises and non-exercises for pregnancy.)

Kitzinger, Sheila. *Experience of Childbirth.* New York: Penguin Books, 1962.
(An introduction to prepared childbirth, with a special psychological approach.)

Walton, Vicki. *Have It Your Way.* New York: Bantam Books, 1978.
(Choices and alternatives for hospital deliveries.)

CAESAREAN BIRTH

Donovan, Bonnie. *The Caesarean Experience.* Boston: Beacon Press, 1977.
(A practical guide for caesarean births.)

NUTRITION

Goldbeck, Nikki. *As You Eat, So Your Baby Grows.* New York: Ceres Press, 1977.
(A short guide to nutrition in pregnancy.)

Turner, Mary and James. *Making Your Own Babyfood.* New York: Bantam Books, 1973.
(A guide to good nutrition.)

BREAST FEEDING

Eiger, Marvin and Sally Olds. *The Complete Book of Breastfeeding.* New York: Bantam Books, 1973.
(A comprehensive guide to breast feeding.)

Ewy, Roger and Donna. *Preparation For Breastfeeding.* New York: Doubleday, 1975.
(A guide to breast feeding.)

CHILDCARE
Fraiberg, Selma. *Every Child's Birthright: In Defense of Mothering.* New York: Basic Books, 1977.
(An investigation of day-care centers and baby nurses, versus nurturing by the mother.)

Levy, Janine. *The Baby Exercise Book.* New York: Pantheon, 1975.
(How to exercise with your baby.)

Marzallo, Jean. *Nine Months, One Day, One Year.* Colophon Books, 1977.
(Pregnancy and birth described by parents.)

Salk, Lee. *What Every Child Would Like His Parents To Know.* New York: David McKay Co., 1972.
(Discussion of a child's everyday feelings and how to handle them.)

CHILD DEVELOPMENT
Brazelton, T. Berry. *Infants and Mothers.* New York: Delta, 1970.
(A guide for parents to early childhood problems.)

———. *Toddlers and Parents.* New York: Delta, 1976.
(A guide for parents to the problems of toddlers.)

Fraiberg, Selma. *The Magic Years.* New York: Scribner and Co., 1959.
(An excellent description of the development of a child.)

Klaus, Marshall and John Kennel. *Maternal and Infant Bonding.* St. Louis, Mo.: Mosby, 1976.
(The importance of early parent-infant attachment.)

Rakowitz, Elly and Gloria Rubin. *Living With Your New Baby.* New York: Franklin Watts, 1978.
(A practical guide for new parents.)

THE SINGLE PARENT
Hope, Karol and Nancy Young. *Momma: The Source Book For Single Mothers.* New York: New American Library, 1976.
(A collection of articles on single parents.)

Klein, Carole. *The Single Parent Experience.* New York: Avon Books, 1973.
(Individual accounts of experiences of single parents.)

OTHER BOOKS OF SPECIAL INTEREST

Bernard, Jessie. *The Future of Motherhood.* New York: Penguin Books, 1975.
(A serious investigation by a sociologist who looks at the roles of women in the family.)

Bing, Elisabeth and Libby Colman. *Making Love During Pregnancy.* New York: Noonday Press, a division of Farrar, Straus and Giroux, 1989.
(An illustrated guide for expectant and new parents.)

The Boston Women's Health Book Collective. *Ourselves and Our Children.* New York: Random House, 1978.
(A thorough look at what it is really like to be parents at all stages of the life cycle and under various family circumstances.)

Keniston, Kenneth. *All Our Children.* New York: Harcourt, Brace and Jovanovich, 1978.
(The Carnegie Report on the American family under stress.)

Whelan, Elizabeth. *A Baby . . . Maybe.* New York: Bobbs-Merrill, 1976.
(Information on making a responsible decision about parenthood.)

Two important books have been published since *Having a Baby After 30* first came out:

Black, Robin J. R. *Prenatal Tests.* New York: Vintage Books, 1988.

Rothman, Barbara Katz. *The Tentative Pregnancy: Prenatal Diagnosis and the Future of Motherhood.* New York: Viking, 1986.

Index

Age 30, 5
Aging, physiological factors of, 16
Alternative Birth Centers, 52, 53, 54
Amniocentesis, 18–21
  risk in, 20
Anemia, 22
Aristotle, 38
Arthritis, 23
Attachment, 63

Baby nurse, 75
Babysitter, 124, 138, 142
Backache, 23
Barbano, Helen, 17
Bibliography, 167–70
Bing, Elisabeth, ix, 151–60
Bing, Peter, 161–64
Birth(s), 51–60
  and early days with baby, 51–77
  as a rite of passage, 57
Birth Control, 2
Body strap, 85
Bonding, 60, 63
Boredom, 128
Brazelton, Barry, 63
Breast feeding, 78–89
  anxieties related to, 84
  duration of, 86
  foreplay, 79
  as a supplement, 83

Business woman, as mother, 134–35

Caesarean births, 25, 26–27, 57, 60, 69, 79
  anesthesia, types of, 27
  incisions, types of, 27
  local anesthetics in, 79
Cardio-vascular disease, 23
Career(s), 7–8
  demands, 117
Change, accepting, 107–08
Check-ups, regular, 24
Childbearing, delayed, 1–29
  fertility-related issues, 15–17
  medical considerations, 13–29
  negative reasons for, 11–13
  phenomenon of, 1–6
  positive reasons for, 6–11
  trend towards, 3
  by whom and why, 6–13
Childbirth
  education, 52, 54, 110, 154
  preparation for, 58
Childcare, adequate, 131
Childcare home, licensed, 124
Children, having more, 147–149
Chromosome #21, 18
Chromosomes, dysfunction in, 17

INDEX

Colman, Libby, ix, 165–66
Colostrum, 79
Complaints, minor, 23
Constipation, 23
Contraceptive(s), xiii
   information, 2

D&C. *See* Dilatation and curettage
Day-care center, 124
Delivery at home, 54
Demands, unavoidable, 141
Depression, 93–108
   loss as a cause of, 106
Diabetes, 23
Diaphragm, 2
Diet, nutritious, 24
Dilatation and curettage, 153
Down's Syndrome, 17–18, 152

Early days with baby, 67–77
Eclampsia, 24
   advanced, 26
Ecology, 11
Economics, 13
Environment, family-centered, 53–54

Fallopian tubes, 16
Father, 109–21
Fathering
   another style of, 111
   involved, 110
Fatigue, 22–23, 138
Fears and anxieties, 21
Fertility, decline of, 16
Fetus malformation(s), 17–21
   possible age-related causes of, 17
Fibroids, 16
First months, concerns of, 78–108
Follicles, 16
Foundation for Medical Research, 14
Fourth trimester, 155
Freedom, 13

Grandparents, 73
Guilt, of working mothers, 131
Guttmacher, Alan, 2

Hay, Sylvia, 17
Hormonal stimulation, 21
Hospital stay, 76
Hotlines, 101, 108
Housekeeper, 74, 124
   full-time, 138

Identity crisis, 103–06
Infections, 16
Infertility, causes of, 15
Inflation, 9
Isolation, sense of, 42, 44
Intercourse, frequence of, 16
IUD, 2
   long-term use of, 15

Job status, 13
   and pregnancy, 45
Jobs, avoidable, 141

Kane, Sidney H., 14
Kennel, John, 62
Klaus, Marshall, 62
Kleinfelder's syndrome, 18

La Leche League, 78, 87, 101
Labor
   and birth, 24–27
   preparation for, 24–25
Labor coach, 54
Lamaze, 25, 111
Lifestyle, change in, 31

Making Love During Pregnancy, xiii, 89
Marriage
   new stresses on, 119
   stable relationship in, 13
Maturity, 12
Menopause, 5
Middle class, 7
Miscarriage, 22, 153

INDEX

Mongolism. *See* Down's Syndrome
Mother love, 59, 60
Mothering
  importance of, 133
  and working, 122–46
Mothers, career options for, 124
Mount Sinai Hospital, 154

Nature, root meaning of, xii
Nausea, 23
Nesting-in, 67, 71, 97, 127
Newborn
  continuous contact with, 62
  feelings for, 60–67
Nursing Mother's Council, 87

Older expectant fathers, concerns of, 37–42
Older expectant mothers, concerns of, 42–49
Orgasm, 91
Ova (eggs), 16
Overpopulation, 11

Parental love, 115
Parenthood, fear of, 11
Parenting, shared, 118
Parents
  attitudes toward, 46
  rejection of, 48
Personality problems, underlying, 102–03
Pill, 2
  long-term use of, 15
Pollution, 11
Postpartum, 28–29
  blues, 93–108
  contraception, 28
  coping with new demands, 28–29
  help, 74–75
  menstruation, 28
  period of adjustment, 92
  recovery, 28

Post partum depression
  physiological effects, 94–95
  psychological effects, 102–108
  stress, 95–102
Postponing pregnancy, most common motive for, 9
Pre-eclampsia, 24
Pregnancy, 30–50
  and older expectant parents, 30–36
  other concerns of, 21–24

Readiness, 140
Reik, Theodore, 106
Rh incompatibility, 25–26
Rhogam, 26
Rooming in, 155
Rudolf Steiner School, 163

Security, sense of, 37
Self, sense of, 11
Sex, 89–93
Sex organs and pregnancy, 89–90
Sexual activity, decline of, 16
Sexual problems due to nursing, 90–91
Sloan, Donald, xii
Sonogram, 19
Sperm, 16
Sugar water, 79

Temperature charts for coitus, 153
Toxemia, 23–24
  symptoms of, 23–24
Trisomy 21. *See* Down's syndrome
Turner's Syndrome, 18
Twins
  fraternal, 16
  identical, 16

Uterus, traumas in, 16

Varicose veins, 23

Warmlines, 101, 108
Weaning, 87
Women, and primary responsibility for children, 122
Women's Liberation Movement, 8

Working
 full time, 137–46
 part time, 130–37

Zero population growth, 3